Your Menotype, Your Menopause

Find Your Type and Free Yourself from the Symptoms of Menopause

Angela Stengler, N.D. & Mark Stengler, N.D.

Prentice
Hall Press

Library of Congress Cataloging-in-Publication Data

Stengler, Angela
   Your menotype, your menopause : find your type and free
   yourself from the symptoms of menopause / by Angela Stengler,
   Mark Stengler ; foreword by Tori Hudson.
      p. cm.
   Includes bibliographical references.
   ISBN 0-7352-0254-0
      1. Menopause. 2. Menopause—Alternative treatment. 3. Naturopathy.
   4. Middle aged women—Health and hygiene. 5. Self-care, Health.
   I. Stengler, Mark.

   RG186.S745 2002
   618.1'7506-dc21   2001056037

Acquisitions Editor: *Edward Claflin*
Production Editor: *Jackie Roulette*
Layout/Interior Design: *Dimitra Coroneos*

© 2002 *by* Angela Stengler, N.D. & Mark Stengler, N.D.

Printed in the United States of America

10 9 8 7 6 5 4 3 2 1

The Natural Physician™ is a trademark of Mark Stengler, N.D.
The term "menotype" is a trademark of Mark Stengler, N.D.

This is a reference book based on research by the author, and the ideas, procedures, and suggestions in this book are not intended as a substitute for the medical advice of your personal health professional. All matters regarding your health require medical supervision. Consult your physician before adopting any of the suggestions in this book (whether or not explicitly noted in the text), as well as about any condition that may require diagnosis or medical attention. In addition, the statements made by the author regarding certain products and services represent the opinions of the author alone, and do not constitute a recommendation or endorsement of any product or service by the publisher. The author and publisher disclaim any liability arising directly or indirectly from the use of the book, or of any products mentioned herein.

Trademarks: All brand names and product names used in this book are trade names, service marks, trademarks, or registered trademarks of their respective owners. Prentice Hall Press is not associated with any product or vendor mentioned in this book.

ISBN 0-7352-0254-0

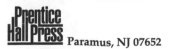 **Paramus, NJ 07652**

http://www.phpress.com

Acknowledgments

We would like to first thank Dr. Tori Hudson for the superb education she provided as our Professor of Gynecology when we were medical students at National College of Naturopathic Medicine. Also to Dr. Donna Guthrie, Dr. Rich Barret, and Dr. Rita Bettenburg. Our thanks to Dr. Marcus Laux for his guidance and words of wisdom. To Ed Claflin and all those at Prentice Hall who made this book possible. Thanks to Jeff Herman, our literary agent. To Dr. Cynthia Robertson and the staff at La Jolla Whole Health Medical Clinic for their support and providing such good service to our patients. Our deepest appreciation to our mothers—Shirley and Mary.

FOREWORD

I first met Angela and Mark Stengler when they were medical students at the National College of Naturopathic Medicine in Portland, Oregon. I remember at that time thinking that they had the intellect, talent, persistence, and commitment to write for publication. I've been impressed over the years since then, that in addition to their private practice, they in fact have taken on many significant projects in order to educate the public on natural medicine.

Naturopathic Physicians occupy a unique position in the medical-care setting because of the scope and diversity of our education. During medical school, the basic and clinical sciences are both included in our training. In addition to that, we receive four years of intense concentration in natural therapeutic practices, including nutrition, nutritional supplementation, herbal medicine, homeopathy, psychotherapy, manipulation, and physical therapies. We also explore conventional therapies, such as pharmaceutical prescriptions, and we learn the indications for chemotherapy, radiation, and surgeries.

As a result, the complete education of a Naturopathic Physician is the most eclectic, in-depth training offered in any medical school, embracing the whole continuum of therapies in alternative and conventional medicine. With this kind of medical training, Naturopathic Physicians understand more clearly the strengths and weaknesses of each type of therapy that we may be called upon to use in any given clinical situation.

For the menopausal woman who seeks medical help, the resources of a Naturopathic Physician offer a much broader range of choices. Doctors like Angela and Mark can give each woman what she needs to assist her in her current symptomatic state, and provide her with prevention strategies for the future.

A naturopathic approach to menopause is unique because it recognizes the importance of each *individual* woman. This is not a "one-size-fits-all" approach. A Naturopathic Physician is not going to prescribe hormone replacement therapy (HRT) for all women, or even for most.

Rather, each physician will make an individualized assessment. A woman is treated according to her particular menopause symptom picture.

For the Naturopathic Physician, no picture is complete until we evaluate a woman's risks for menopause-related conditions such as uterine prolapse, osteoporosis, heart disease, and Alzheimer's disease, as well as the risks of other conditions such as macular degeneration and colon cancer. Once the assessment and evaluation have been done, therapeutic plans and interventions can be chosen from the whole spectrum of possibilities—exercise, counseling, nutrition, nutritional supplementation, herbs, homeopathy, natural hormones, and conventional hormones. And we may recommend other pharmaceuticals for conditions such as osteoporosis, high blood pressure, and high cholesterol.

Creating an organized and effective model to deal with so many variables requires a great deal of knowledge about menopause and a great deal of knowledge about all the many therapies. Angela and Mark have created a highly effective tool to assist in this process. Understanding your "menopause type" can clearly help you sort through many options and select what is the best approach for *your* situation.

Your Menotype, Your Menopause is the result of the Stenglers' combined knowledge and their many years of education and clinical experience. Their expertise has helped many women find their way through the maze of many menopause symptoms and therapies. Using natural, plant-based healing—as well as judicious use of natural hormones, conventional hormones, and selected pharmaceuticals—these doctors help make it easier and safer for women to more effectively manage their menopause.

Many menopause books have been published, but the depth and breadth of *Your Menotype, Your Menopause* and the practical well-founded recommendations make this book a necessary selection for every woman's home health library and a resource for both alternative and conventional practitioners.

Tori Hudson, N.D.
Author of *Women's Encyclopedia of Natural Medicine,*
Professor at the National College of Naturopathic Medicine, and
Medical Director of A Woman's Time (a woman's integrative
     health clinic in Portland, Oregon)

CONTENTS

3
NATURE'S TOP HERBAL HORMONE BALANCERS   53

4
CUSTOMIZING YOUR HORMONE REPLACEMENT   79

7
HOMEOPATHY   133

8
EXERCISE   141

9
PUTTING IT ALL TOGETHER   161

10
HEART DISEASE AND MENOPAUSE   177

11
BONES OF STEEL   199

12
NATURAL SOLUTIONS TO COMMON FEMALE CONDITIONS 215

$\mathcal{I}$NTRODUCTION: DISCOVERING CHOICES

Menopause can be a confusing time in a woman's life. Whether its symptoms are mild or severe, many or few, it will certainly bring challenges.

If you've been trying to find a single doctor, book, or authority that can bring you up to date on your treatment options—both pharmaceutical and natural—to cope with those challenges, you're probably discouraged by all the lack of agreement among experts as to which treatments are best.

Talking with your medical doctor or reading a brochure produced by a pharmaceutical company might lead you to conclude that hormone replacement therapy (HRT) is the only logical choice for a woman experiencing menopause. On the other hand, if you consult with a "holistic" doctor, nutritionist, or chiropractor, you might think that natural therapies are the *only* way to go.

In fact, either approach can be an acceptable option, depending upon an individual's symptom profile—what we call her "menotype." Though I favor natural treatments, I also have an extensive background in conventional medicine, and I would certainly recommend HRT when it's appropriate. However, I part with the mainstream medical community in that I don't believe any doctor should prescribe HRT as a universal "panacea" for the symptoms of menopause.

Hormone replacement therapy (HRT) first became popular as a medical treatment in the 1960s, but it has actually been around for thousands of years. In ancient Chinese texts, there are descriptions of elders who rejuvenate their sex lives by drinking the urine of teenage boys and girls. (The urine contains hormones.) In traditional Chinese medicine, some doctors would add the placenta (afterbirth) of a newborn to soup or make it into pills, which is another form of hormone therapy.

While both practices may sound strange, the sources of hormones have often been unusual—including the present-day practice of giving Premarin® to menopausal women. Premarin® is estrogen derived from the urine of pregnant mares—unwilling donors who are kept in tight stalls throughout their pregnancy.

Historically, estrogen was first isolated from the urine of pregnant women in 1923. Although pharmaceutical companies were interested in this female sex hormone, it wasn't commercially viable to produce estrogen from this particular source. It was not until 1943 that researchers began the practice of extracting estrogen from pregnant mares' urine. The patents for this horse-urine estrogen extract were sold to Ayerst Laboratories.

The biggest boost for Premarin® came in 1966, when gynecologist Robert Wilson, M.D., published the book *Feminine Forever*. Heavily promoted by Ayerst Laboratories, the book was essentially a promotional piece for Premarin®. In his book, Dr. Wilson stated that menopause was a disease resulting from estrogen deficiency and could therefore be treated by addressing this deficiency.

Dr. Wilson also made it clear that estrogen deficiency was a problem unique to females. In his view, low levels of female hormones led directly to a sexless life, which would inevitably spiral downward. As suggested by the book's title, Dr. Wilson represented that the magic pill Premarin® would restore a woman's femininity and help her maintain her youth.

Feminine Forever was distributed to doctors' offices via pharmaceutical sales representatives, and excerpts appeared in many women's magazines. By 1975, more than 6 million American women were taking the drug. Later, however, when doctors found that continuous use of Premarin® substantially increased the risk of endometrial cancer, they altered their approach and started to prescribe it in conjunction with Provera®, a synthetic version of progesterone. This modification appeared to lower the rate of endometrial cancers. However, as I'll be pointing out later in this book, Provera® has its own list of potential side effects.

If that isn't confusing enough, a study published in *The Journal of the American Medical Association* in 2000 found that postmenopausal women who use the combined regimen of estrogen and progestin (synthetic hormones) have a relatively higher risk of breast cancer than women who take only estrogen. The postmenopausal women who used this combination of synthetic estrogen and progesterone during the prior four years had a 40-percent higher risk for these cancers than women who had never used hormone replacement therapy.

Given all the problems and risks that come with HRT, you might well wonder why pharmaceutical companies have never taken a closer look at alternative treatments, such as herbal extracts and other natural remedies, including natural hormones. The economics of the pharmaceutical industry makes such a research investment impossible. No one can patent a substance found in nature. Without a patent, a company cannot corner the market on a product and control its price. So even if a natural product is safer and more effective than a prescription drug, no pharmaceutical company has an incentive to promote it.

It would be unfair to look only at the risks associated with HRT without also examining its benefits. For example, even if synthetic estrogen raises a woman's risk of cancer, pharmaceutical companies claim that it will also protect her against heart disease. That's an important claim. Heart disease kills more women each year than any other medical condition. In the United States alone, it kills an estimated 250,000 women.

It's true that synthetic estrogen replacement has been shown to reduce many of the "markers" associated with heart disease—that is, measurable factors such as cholesterol, homocysteine, and fibrinogen that indicate whether a woman has a low or high risk of heart disease. But if even these markers have lower readings, do you really have greater protection from cardiovascular disease?

Conventional practitioners routinely state that hormone replacement therapy reduces the risk of a heart attack by approximately 40% to 50%, a statistic based on several epidemiological studies.

However, some factors are often overlooked when this impressive statistic is offered. First, women who take estrogen are more likely to enjoy a higher economic status, better diet and healthier lifestyle, and access to better healthcare. They're also less likely to smoke. These contributing factors have not been taken into account when assessing the data on heart disease and hormone replacement therapy.

Also the 1998 HERS (Heart and Estrogen/Progestin Replacement Study) was designed to record the incidence of mortality among 2,700 postmenopausal women who had coronary artery disease. The study showed that taking hormones did not reduce their risk of death. In fact, if we look at the statistics of this study, they indicate that women who undergo hormone replacement using synthetic hormones are more likely to die in the first year after menopause than are women who *don't* take the hormones! It should come as no surprise that the American Heart Association recently issued a report stating that "There are insufficient data to suggest that HRT should be initiated for the sole purpose of primary prevention of CVD [cardiovascular disease]."

Given all of the current evidence, it seems to me that there are far better ways to reduce your risk of heart disease with the methods you'll find in this book—including exercise; diet; supplements such as garlic, vitamin E, B vitamins, and other antioxidants; stress reduction; and other techniques.

Advocates of hormone replacement will also argue that estrogen protects against osteoporosis. Again, this is an important claim, as an estimated one in two women over age 50 will develop osteoporosis in her lifetime. Nearly half of all women over the age of 65 are likely to suffer fractures as a result of osteoporosis.

Synthetic estrogen has been shown to decrease fracture rate. I do believe, based on studies that have been done on estrogen, that the hormone has a protective effect and can help preserve bone density. However, we also know that estrogen is only one factor in the osteoporosis equation. Many researchers feel that progesterone increases bone density, as do other hormones such as testosterone.

Lifestyle also plays a major role. Smoking and excess alcohol increase the risk for osteoporosis. Exercise and a healthy diet, on the other hand, can strengthen bones. Supplements such as calcium, magnesium, vitamin D, and others are very important, and the supplement ipriflavone is one of the few substances shown to increase bone density when used in conjunction with calcium. None of these supplements carries the risk of cancer. And as you will learn, the beginnings of osteoporosis actually begin many years before menopause.

It really all comes down to individualized treatment. You need what is best for you and your situation—and to discover that, you need to note your own symptoms and discover your menotype, be open to different therapies, and then see how you respond to those therapies.

That's what this book will help you do.

Angela Stengler, N.D.
Mark Stengler, N.D.

1

$\mathscr{T}$HE MENOTYPE SOLUTION

$\mathscr{H}$ave you ever thought about what the term "menopause" actually means? Most of us invest the word with lots of emotion, and no wonder. Menopausal women are often portrayed in movies as nightmarishly neurotic or uncontrollably hysterical. And, of course, menopause signals the end of our childbearing years, a change that can stir all kinds of confusing feelings within us. The word itself derives from the Latin root *meno,* meaning "month," and the Greek word *pauo,* meaning "to make cease." In medical terms, it simply means the permanent cessation of menstruation.

Here's what most of us know: It's a natural, normal stage in the cycle of every woman's life. Deep down, we're well aware that it won't turn us into quivering masses of hysteria. That only happens in the movies. And while it's a big change, every woman goes through it. It's normal and it's natural. So why does the very thought of it make us so uncomfortable?

Here are some possible reasons:

Hot flashes
Night sweats
Insomnia
Depression
Fatigue
Irritability
Mood swings
Anxiety

Memory loss
Inability to concentrate
Vaginal dryness
Vaginal atrophy (thinning)
Urinary problems
   (incontinence or urinary
   tract infections)
Skin changes

Headaches	Acne
Joint pain	Increase in facial hair
Heart palpitations	Hair loss from the scalp
Low sex drive	

The truth is that menopause is a time of profound transition, during which hormones and metabolic processes change. These changes are what cause all of those symptoms. But while most women will experience some of the symptoms listed above, they can also learn how to lessen them and maintain a strong and happy quality of life.

THE MEDIEVAL MENOPAUSE MINDSET

I remember watching my own mother struggle through her menopause when I was a teenager. Her doctor wanted to put her on hormones, but she respectfully refused his advice. In fact, she never took anything for her symptoms. She didn't want pharmaceuticals, and, at the time, she didn't have access to information about effective natural therapies. The result was that she went through a lot of needless suffering.

Today, thankfully, the situation has changed. A lot more information is available on various ways to treat the symptoms of menopause. Even if you're like my mother and shy away from pharmaceuticals, healthcare providers can offer many highly effective natural treatments that will relieve discomfort and put bounce back into your life. We should be leaping for joy!

Unfortunately, many conventional doctors haven't yet heard the good news and are still living in the dark ages as far as menopause is concerned. If you're now having symptoms and seeing a conventional doctor about them, you know what I mean. He or she has probably explained to you no more about menopause than "it's an estrogen-deficiency problem." In other words, it's a condition resulting from a shortage of one particular hormone. That's pretty much the same information they gave to my mother.

UNWELCOME SURPRISES

Many of the women who come to my clinic are confused by what's happening to their bodies—and no wonder! "Why am I crying so much?" one woman asks me. "I don't feel any pain. I'm not unhappy. I just feel all weepy sometimes!"

Some have temporary memory loss, which can be frightening. "I need to write things down," a woman told me. "I feel like my memory doesn't work any more."

Some women experience depressed libido. "Those times when we could hardly wait to climb into bed together? That seems like ancient history," said Marianne. It just seemed "unfair," she told me, that menopause came so early and put such a damper on her sex life. "You want to know the truth? Sex is one of the last things on my mind." She went on to describe what had happened to her libido. She'd always had an active and satisfying sex life. Now, sex was the last thing on her mind.

Then there are the infamous hot flashes. Cynthia, a woman in her late 40's, observed, "I used to get cold very easily. Now I get hot flashes and night sweats. I don't dare to dress as warmly as I used to, because I'll end up feeling stuffy, overheated, and sweaty. And you should see me at night. It's a regular tug of war! I'm always throwing the covers off—and my husband keeps trying to drag them back on."

Whatever your symptoms, you're unlikely to be satisfied with an oversimplistic explanation like "estrogen deficiency" that ignores the confusion and anxiety you may be feeling. If your doctor can't do better, then it may be time to seek a new healthcare provider to help you through the challenges of menopause.

THE ONE-SIZE-FITS-ALL APPROACH

If the problem is that simple, then so is the solution: Replace the deficient estrogen, and perhaps throw in a pinch of the complementary hormone progesterone for good measure. This approach certainly seems to help some women, but is it always really in their best interest?

Menopausal women are often told that hormone replacement may carry some risks—among them, the increased possibility of getting certain cancers. But the benefits of hormone replacement are so numerous—at least according to many doctors—that it's well worth doing. They'll tell you it can help prevent your having a heart attack; can reduce the rate of bone loss from osteoporosis; and might even help stave off Alzheimer's disease and colon cancer.

Some women, however, continue to wonder about the safety and effectiveness of a therapy that replaces the body's natural hormones with extracts of hormones from farm animals.

Yes, animals.

Premarin®, the most widely prescribed hormone in the world, comes from horse urine. So is it any wonder that one of my patients recently asked, incredulously, "Can it really be *good* for me?"

Some medical doctors believe it *is* good for you, mostly because they're used to treating injuries and diseases. That's what they're trained to do, and that's what they do best. So when a patient comes to a clinic looking for help, it's only natural for her doctor to treat her condition as a disease. The doctor sees his mission clearly: Make a diagnosis, then administer the right medication. If her symptoms disappear, he has done his job.

The problem, of course, is that menopause is not a disease, but a natural event that occurs in the life of every woman; and women going through it don't need a cure—they need guidance and relief. Besides, it's inaccurate and much too simplistic to say that menopause is caused by an estrogen deficiency. In fact, progesterone levels drop dramatically, and other hormones also fluctuate dramatically—including Pregnenlone, DHEA, and testosterone.

In any case, even if hormone levels do go into sharp decline, why should doctors assume that elevating them is an appropriate treatment? Men as well as women seem to have more difficulty metabolizing hormones as they get older. If that's so, then the reduction in hormone levels may actually be an advantage. After all, women are at greater risk of breast and uterine cancers when hormone levels are elevated. Perhaps this is the body's way of protecting itself against hormone-induced cancers.

While I think there is a place for hormone replacement therapy—especially using natural hormones—I don't think we should assume that a woman's body is somehow "coming up short" during menopause. And I do believe that medicine has gone too far with the notion that hormone replacement is the solution for all women.

TAKING THE ALTERNATIVE ROUTE

Unlike my mother's generation, women who reject hormone replacement today don't have to sit back and suffer through their symptoms without relief. Many turn to the "natural route," using herbal or homeopathic remedies to reduce their discomfort. Many also make nutritional changes, adding soy foods and protein powder, as well as vitamin E (for heart protection) and calcium (to protect the bones) to their diet. A few even try using progesterone cream or some other kind of "natural hormone replacement."

It makes sense that women prefer to use the least invasive, most effective therapy available to get relief, but are they really as effective as hormone replacement? And what about reducing the risk of the more serious effects of menopause, such as osteoporosis?

Although many conventional practitioners still contend that natural therapies are unproven or unscientific, a plethora of studies have been done that show otherwise, and physicians in other parts of the world who commonly prescribe natural therapies get excellent results with their patients. German doctors, for example, often advise women to use the herb Black Cohosh to relieve their menopausal symptoms. Both thorough research and the gratitude of German women bear witness to the effectiveness of this approach.

But what about bone loss? Some women assume from what they've heard that estrogen replacement prevents osteoporosis, but that's not accurate. Most studies show that estrogen replacement slows the rate at which bone cells are lost, but it doesn't necessarily help you build bone. Some alternative treatments also halt bone loss, but some actually *build* bone. This is important because the process of bone loss begins to occur many years before menopause, in the early 20's or earlier.

Again, none of this is to say that there is no place for hormone replacement therapy in the treatment of menopausal symptoms. Clearly there is. But it's not for everyone. Whether you're inclined to use conventional hormone replacement or to take the natural route, you need knowledge to make a wise and informed judgment. Remember, knowledge is power! So let's start by taking a closer look at menopause to come to a better understanding of how it works and what it does. Then we'll look at a unique way of tailoring a program especially for YOU!

WHAT HAPPENS AT THE ONSET OF MENOPAUSE

Make no mistake about it, some tremendous physiological changes occur during menopause.

In simplest terms, menopause is a transitional time—a progression from the stage of life when your ovaries regularly release eggs on a monthly basis to a new stage of life when your ovaries will no longer release any eggs at all. During that transition, there's a major shift in the cycles of hormone production. The ovarian production of the hormones estrogen and progesterone goes into sharp decline. In response, your brain begins to release increasing amounts of two other hormones that go by the initials FSH and LH. This is a final attempt to stimulate the ovaries to start releasing eggs again.

Other changes occur as well. As egg production slows and finally comes to a halt, the uterus no longer sheds its lining on a monthly basis. Menstruation ceases. Your body will still produce estrogen, progesterone, and other hormones, but the supply comes from new areas—specifically, mostly from the adrenal glands, which are located on top of each kidney, and from fat tissue.

You may end up with a shortage of testosterone, which may affect libido and bone density, and may influence heart health as well. Your thyroid gland may become sluggish, forcing your body's energy-burning power into decline and possibly also contributing to fatigue, depression, dry skin, lowered immunity, and constipation.

There may be still other changes. Some women have elevated cholesterol during menopause. Osteoporosis may accelerate, leaving you with fragile bones that fracture easily.

Some of these changes are totally internal, so it's hard to see their effects, but we know that menopausal women are more likely to suffer from a wide range of health problems that seem directly related to the physical and hormonal changes that are taking place.

DIFFERENT VIEWS OF THE MATTER

Hormonal changes aren't the only factors that influence the way we experience menopause. The culture we live in also has a profound effect.

In North America, our culture demeans menopause. We treat it as a midlife crisis—a time when a woman falls under the control of hormone imbalances, resulting in wacky behavior.

This isn't the view held in many other places around the world. In some societies, menopause is viewed as a sign of wisdom and maturity, and women going through it are held in deep respect. Does that make a difference? Research shows that menopausal women who are treated more respectfully do not experience the strong symptoms that we see among women in industrialized nations. In fact, one study found that rural Mayan Indians going through menopause showed *none* of the symptoms we typically associate with it. Their monthly menstruation ceased, of course, but these women never experienced hot flashes or showed any signs of osteoporosis. Diet and exercise certainly played a role, but researchers found that cultural attitudes also had a tremendous impact.

Mayan women weren't the only ones to show this effect. Women in China and Japan also seem particularly immune to the severe symptoms of menopause that are generally experienced by women in America (unless they move here and switch to our diet and lifestyle habits), and again societal attitudes proved as important as diet and exercise.

If there's a message in this, it's pretty straightforward. If you see your menopause as a coming of age and a maturing into greater calmness and wisdom, you're far more likely to experience it in a positive way.

THE MAIN STAGES OF MENOPAUSE

The menopausal transition usually starts between the ages of 48 and 52. Seventy-five percent of menopausal women experience hot flashes for about two years, but another 25 percent keep having them for five years or more. A few women continue to have hot flashes up to 16 years after menopause began.

If menopause still lies ahead of you, take a look at other women in your immediate family, especially those in your maternal line, to estimate when it will begin. If your mother and her mother (maternal grandmother) experienced an early menopause, then it is more likely that you will as well. The opposite is also true: If they experienced a late menopause, then chances are greater that you will experience a later menopause. This is a probability, not a certainty, however. And if you are significantly overweight (10 to 20 percent over your "ideal" weight), you increase your chances of having a later menopause.

Perimenopause—sometimes called premenopause—is the first of the three main stages of menopause and usually starts a year or two before the onset of full-blown menopausal symptoms. This is the time when the menstrual cycle begins to change. The ovaries no longer release eggs consistently. Progesterone levels drop. Your periods become irregular.

Even in perimenopause, you may have hot flashes and other symptoms. Though the span of this stage is usually just a year or two, a few women may start perimenopause when they're in their 30's—long before the second stage begins.

The second stage of the transition is *menopause* itself. During this time, hormones decline sharply, your periods stop, and you'll develop all the symptoms you're going to have.

The third and final stage is *postmenopause*. Many women express health concerns about this stage, and justifiably so. This is the time when they will be at greater risk for osteoporosis, cancer, Alzheimer's disease, and osteoarthritis.

PREMATURE MENOPAUSE

There's no such thing as the "average" menopause experience. Some women begin to go through it long before the age of 50. Premature menopause is defined as the cessation of menses before the age of 40. At the onset of premature menopause, ovulation stops, hormone levels drop, and the woman has no more menstrual cycles.

The medical literature states that about one out of every 100 women in the United States is likely to experience premature menopause. In two-thirds of these cases, doctors can't figure out why it happens, but for the remaining cases, there's a known, medical reason. Likely causes include severe infections of the reproductive tract (which can damage ovarian structures), genetic abnormalities, systemic disease, lack of blood flow to the ovaries, cigarette smoking, excessive exposure to radiation, chemotherapy drugs, early puberty, major life stressors, and surgeries that impair blood flow to the ovaries.

Of course, you're certain to have premature menopause if your ovaries are surgically removed. (Since surgery induces the early onset of menopausal symptoms, this kind is often referred to as "artificial menopause.") Removing both ovaries is referred to as bilateral oophorectomy. Sometimes this procedure is done to prevent the spread of tumors of the ovaries, uterus, or breasts. In other cases, women who have endometriosis can benefit from ovarian surgery.

Some surgeons remove the ovaries while performing a hysterectomy (uterus removal). The three most common reasons for hysterectomy are uterine fibroids, endometriosis, and uterine prolapse.

Once the ovaries are removed, the symptoms of menopause occur quite rapidly unless hormone replacement is began

BE KIND TO YOURSELF

As you probably know, the physiological changes that occur at menopause make up only a part of the picture. Emotional changes can present an even greater challenge. Medical doctors—especially male medical doctors—may encourage their patients to ignore the flood tides of feelings that may occur and just deal with physical symptoms. In my opinion, those doctors are as wrong as they can be.

Menopause can be confusing, stressful, and even frightening. If women need anything at this point in their lives, it's reassurance. When my own patients begin to experience the early signs of perimenopause, the first thing I want to say is, "Take a deep breath, and tell yourself everything is going to be all right."

Because it is.

THE SEVEN STEPS TO SUCCESSFUL COPING

Menopause is, in every sense, a transition that will take its own time. But there are ways to make it a good, productive time. Try following these steps.

- **Make a plan.** After seeing so many women in my practice go through menopause over the years, I began to notice that each woman fell into one of several typical symptom profiles, which we call "menotypes." This book will help you discover and develop an optimal plan for your unique menotype.

- **Pay attention to what you are feeling.** Your symptoms are a guide to what is going on with your body.

- **Educate yourself.** Learn everything you can about the process of menopause so that it won't seem such a mystery to you.

- **Get the right help.** If you haven't already done so, choose an integrative doctor who will listen to you and will help you stay as healthy as possible. Depending on your needs, you might want to consult with a number of health practitioners, including a nutritionist, chiropractor, counselor, or better yet, a naturopathic doctor, who is trained to assess your symptoms and help you in the most comprehensive way.

- **Give your lifestyle a face-lift.** Alter your habits as much as necessary to maintain optimum health and minimize menopausal symptoms. For example, if you don't exercise, now is the time to get on a regular program. If you smoke, do whatever is necessary to quit. If your diet needs improvement, start working on it right away. Now is the time!

🕊 **Improve your spiritual health.** Recent health studies point to the inescapable conclusion that people who have fulfilling spiritual lives are more likely to remain healthy and energetic in their later years. With spiritual nurture, people also bounce back more quickly from disease and they are likely to live longer.

🕊 **Set future goals for yourself.** You can make some important lifestyle choices right now that will help you feel more fulfilled in every way. What is important to you? What do you want to do that excites and fulfills you?

INTRODUCING THE MENOTYPES

To help you find out as quickly and easily as possible what menopause treatments are most likely to be helpful to you, it's helpful to recognize that symptoms tend to fall into certain patterns. These patterns are so universal that I have "coined" them "menotypes."

Knowing what your own menotype is will help you find your way comfortably through the transition of menopause. It will also put information at your fingertips that can help your healthcare provider accurately assess your needs and put together the best, most well-rounded program that will work for you as an individual.

For each of the three basic menotypes described in this book, there are certain specific, menopausal symptoms you can identify by yourself or with the help of a physician or health practitioner. Each of these menotypes also has certain risk factors associated with it. I'll recommend a specific approach for each menotype—just as I do for my patients—to help make menopause easier for you and to reduce your associated health risks as much as possible.

The first thing you need to do in determining your menotype is to take a close look at what's happening to you physically and emotionally.

Based on your self-evaluation, you'll be able to make the initial determination about whether your type is m-A, m-B, or m-C.

To a lesser degree you can assess what your menotype will be even before you enter menopause. If your mother and grandmother have told you that they had a very hard time when they were going through menopause, then there's a higher chance your own type will be m-B or m-C. If you have had your ovaries removed, then you automatically know that you would do best on the m-C program.

If you are a healthy woman and have no signs of osteoporosis, you may be more likely to fall into the m-A or m-B categories. We often find that women who have suffered from severe premenstrual syndrome (PMS) are more likely to have a more difficult time with menopause so they're more likely to be m-B or m-C types.

But these are generalizations. Most of us don't know what menopause is going to be like until we begin to go through it. Since the obvious symptoms are only part of the story, I recommend that you get a full medical assessment to help you form a complete and full picture of your menotype profile. In addition to getting a measurement of hormone levels (preferably, with the saliva test I will be describing in this book), I also recommend getting a bone density measurement.

A PAUSE FOR SOME HISTORY

How much attention have you paid to your health in the past?

The answer to that question can be surprisingly relevant to your experience with menopause. For example, if you have been a heavy smoker and coffee drinker, you have increased your risk of getting osteoporosis—and that will negatively affect your menotype profile.

On the other hand, if you have taken very good care of yourself by maintaining a healthful diet, exercising regularly, and using stress-reduction techniques, you've already affected your profile in a positive way!

Despite these generalizations, it's important to note that your past lifestyle, health history, and family history do not *guarantee* what menotype category you will be in. I have seen women who had a model lifestyle, with no significant family history of menopause problems, who needed the therapies recommended for the most severe profile.

If you're already in midmenopause, you can still get many benefits from identifying your menotype. You may find that you're doing more than is necessary to reduce your current symptoms. On the other hand, you may learn that some nagging problems you've been experiencing can be quite easily solved. Once they begin using appropriate therapies, many women find that their joints ache less and they become more mobile, their depression lifts and their mood improves, their libido and energy increase, and their body weight becomes easier to manage without drastic dieting.

TESTING, TESTING

There are some tests every woman should take when assessing her menotype. Here are some brief summaries of what they are and what they do.

Bloodwork

- *FSH*—pituitary hormone is elevated at time of menopause
- *CBC*—complete blood count to look for anemia and to make sure the immune cells are normal
- *Chemistry profile*—looks at many things including glucose, electrolytes, and liver enzymes
- *Thyroid panel (include TSH and free T3)*—evaluates thyroid function

Other

- *Cardiovascular profile*—should include counts for total cholesterol, HDL (good cholesterol), LDL (bad cholesterol), triglycerides, Apolipoprotein A-1 (Apo A-1), Apolipoprotein B, homocysteine, fibrinogen, Lipoprotein A (Lp(a)), C-Reactive Protein, Ferritin, Insulin
- *Saliva Hormone Testing*—should include estrone, estradiol, estriol, progesterone, testosterone, DHEA

X-ray

⮞ Bone density (DEXA scan)

I also recommend reviewing your health history with a doctor, preferably one well versed in conventional and natural therapies. A complete physical exam is required to rule out any disease processes. A mammogram may also be needed.

MENOTYPE QUIZ

The menotype quiz is designed to help you target the menotype that best fits you and your menopause experience. Simply go through the symptom list and circle the number that best describes you. Then read over the menotypes at a glance. Finally and most importantly, read the menotype profiles and snapshots that follow. The rest of the book will tell you how to use your new knowledge in coping with the challenges your own menopause brings you.

Rating scale

0—never have this symptom	2—moderate
1—mild	3—severe

Symptom list

Symptom				
Hot flashes (daytime)	0	1	(2)	3
Night sweats	0	1	(2)	3
Insomnia	0	1	2	(3)
Depression	0	1	(2)	3
Anxiety	0	(1)	2	3
Loss of memory	0	1	(2)	3
Vaginal dryness	(0)	1	2	3
Vaginal atrophy (thinning)	0	(1)	2	3
Urinary problems (incontinence or urinary tract infections)	(0)	1	2	3
Low sex drive	0	1	(2)	3
Acne	(0)	1	2	3
Increase in facial hair	(0)	1	2	3
Hair loss (head)	(0)	1	(2)	3

Interpreting your score:

- If most of your symptoms are 0 and 1, then you are likely menotype A (m-A).
- If most of your symptoms are 1 and 2, then you are likely menotype B (m-B).
- If most of your symptoms are 2 and 3, then you are likely menotype C (m-C).

Note: If you have moderate to severe osteoporosis, go to menotype C.

SNAPSHOT: MENOTYPE A

Symptom picture:

- None or mild menopausal symptoms.
- No osteoporosis present. No strong family history of osteoporosis.

Hormone testing:

- Normal to low-normal levels. (See Chapter 4 for more information.)

Treatment recommendations:

- Plant-based diet high in phytoestrogens. High-potency multivitamin, natural vitamin E, and calcium/magnesium supplements. Exercise program.
- Consider homeopathy and/or acupuncture as preventive treatments.
- Herbal therapy is optional.

MENOTYPE PROFILES

Menotype A

Those women who fit the description of m-A have an easier time than the other two groups in deciding which course of action to take because A types really do not experience strong menopausal symptoms such as hot flashes, night sweats, and so on. They do not have any signs of osteoporosis, and neither saliva nor blood hormone analysis show a major deficiency of any of the hormones tested.

Unfortunately, we find the percentage of women who we see in our clinic and who belong to this category is small, about 5–10 percent. Of course women that come to our clinic are seeking help for relief from menopausal symptoms, so are less likely to be menotype A. As we will discuss later, the percentage of women who would fit into this category in other cultures would be much higher, and in some cases, the dominant menotype.

SHE TRIED IT

When her menses stopped three years ago, Betty, at age 56, was concerned about her risk for osteoporosis. At that time, she had occasional irritability and no hot flashes. Betty had always exercised, but her diet was poor (low in vegetables, fruits, whole grains, while high in refined sugars and fast foods). Her bone density was normal as was her most recent mammogram. In addition, her bloodwork showed no elevated markers for heart disease. Betty fit the menotype A category. She began taking a homeopathic remedy for irritability, which helped her feel more balanced emotionally. In addition, I recommended a multivitamin, vitamin E, calcium, and magnesium, and urged Betty to increase the amount of fruits and vegetables in her diet. She had a low risk of osteoporosis, but for safety's sake, we would continue to monitor her bone density in the future. Now, three years later, Betty consistently follows the menotype A program with success.

The goals of menotype A's are to maintain good health, prevent common conditions that tend to come up during menopause (osteoporosis, heart disease), and prevent common menopausal symptoms (such as hot flashes, vaginal dryness, and so on) from occurring.

Plant foods, which are full of naturally occurring phytoestrogens, and especially plants containing sterols, known to have hormone-balancing effects, should form a major part of your diet. Soy, for example, is rich in isoflavones. It helps to reduce hot flashes (although not generally a big problem with menotype A's), reduce cholesterol, and is showing some promise in preventing bone loss. Population studies have shown that fermented soy foods (such as tofu and miso) prevent cancer of the breast, uterus, and other types of the disease. As we'll discuss later on, women in the m-A category who want to be more proactive can also use herbal and nutritional supplements, homeopathic remedies, and acupuncture to help prevent the development of symptoms. And regular exercise, of course, is a great way to help prevent osteoporosis, heart disease, insomnia, and mood changes.

SHE TRIED IT

Sara was a 47-year-old woman suffering from hot flashes and mood swings. She had not had a menstrual cycle for a year, and bloodwork confirmed she was menopausal. The rest of her blood chemistry was normal, as was her bone density scan. Sara exercised only on the weekends. Her diet consisted mainly of pasta, fruit, and diet soda. Because Sara's symptoms were low in intensity and her risk factors were minor, she was a good candidate for the menotype A protocol. Sara, however, made it clear that she was not interested in taking herbs, so instead, I recommended lifestyle changes to improve her condition. Sara committed to exercising four times a week, as well as to increasing her vegetable and water intake. She also agreed to take a multivitamin and protein shake each morning. After two months, she reported her hot flashes had decreased somewhat, and she had quite a bit more energy. Her husband stated she was "easier to live with." Sara felt good about the program I had her on and showed some willingness to be more aggressive with her supplementation program, especially to help decrease her hot flashes. I had Sara take an extra 800 IU of natural vitamin E as well as a soy isoflavone supplement (150 mg). After two months of this expanded program, she reported an 80-percent improvement in her hot flashes and mood swings. Sara felt that her exercise and diet changes made a dramatic improvement. In addition, I felt her positive attitude toward menopause helped her get through this transitional time more effectively. I spoke with Sara another year later and she reported being "done with menopause" and feeling "20 years younger."

Here is a sample program, but be sure to read the rest of the book to tailor an individual program that's right for you.

Menotype-A Sample Program

- ❧ whole food diet (see Chapter 5)
- ❧ high-potency multivitamin (without iron)
- ❧ vitamin E (mixed)—400 IU
- ❧ calcium (daily total of 1000 mg) and magnesium (daily total of 500 mg) or a bone formula containing these and other minerals for bone health (see Chapter 11 for details)
- ❧ condition-specific supplements depending on what is going on with you (for example, ginseng for energy, St. John's Wort for depression, vitamin C for the immune system)
- ❧ regular exercise

NOTE: Cardiovascular-specific supplements are recommended if risk factors are present.

Menotype B

Those who fit the profile of menotype B have more choices to make. They're experiencing some uncomfortable menopausal symptoms, possibly while trying to juggle a career and/or home life. Some say they feel scared, confused, and angry at the same time. They may feel scared because the symptoms they're feeling are stronger than they had anticipated or because they're becoming aware of their increased risk for heart disease and osteoporosis. They may also be frightened they'll get breast cancer, a condition that can appear regardless of menotype.

Confusion and anxiety may arise over deciding which approach to take toward relieving symptoms. A woman might be under pressure from her doctor to use hormone replacement, or she may be unsure if the natural treatment she wants to use actually works.

Some anger may also enter the picture. Her spouse may not be sensitive to the changes and stresses she's going through. While a little joking about the subject is tolerable—some men don't know when to quit—some understanding is required as well. Anger may be directed toward her doctor, as well, who may not be taking her emotional symptoms seriously enough.

~~~~~~

SNAPSHOT: MENOTYPE B

Symptom picture:

- Mild to moderate menopausal symptoms.
- No personal history of osteoporosis.
- Family history of osteoporosis is not a major factor (although could be present).
- If osteoporosis is a major risk factor, then go directly to menotype C.

Hormone testing:

- Normal to borderline low. (See Chapter 4 for more information.)

Treatment recommendations:

- *First line of treatment:* Herbal therapy along with nutritional supplement, diet, and lifestyle recommendations as given for menotype A for 6-8 weeks. If there is no response, go to the second line of treatment described below. Consider homeopathy and/or acupuncture treatment.
- *Second line of treatment:* Natural progesterone and/or DHEA or Pregnenelone use. If vaginal dryness and/or severe hot flashes/night sweats are present and do not respond to treatment in menotype B recommendations, then use natural hormone replacement as described in menotype C.

A little more thought must be given when deciding what approach is best for women in this group. In our experience, this represents the largest menotype group, making up approximately 50–60 percent of menopausal women we see.

Menopausal symptoms of menotype B are generally rated in the mild to moderate category. For some women in this group, symptoms are slight, such as the occasional hot flash, mild insomnia, or a reduction in libido. For others, the symptoms are so pronounced that they interfere with daily activities.

As with menotype A's, diet is very important in the prevention of chronic illnesses such as heart disease, cancer, and many others. However, my experience has been that diet alone does not usually make a pronounced impact on the menopausal symptoms of m-B's.

MENOTYPES AT A GLANCE

Menotype A
- Little to no menopausal symptoms.
- No signs of osteoporosis.
- Ovaries have not been removed.
- Normal decrease in menopausal hormone levels.

Menotype B
- Mild to moderate menopausal symptoms.
- Normal bone density or beginning of osteoporosis.
- Ovaries have not been removed.
- Mild to moderate decrease in menopausal hormone levels.

Menotype C
- Severe menopausal symptoms.
- Moderate to severe osteoporosis.
- Ovaries have been removed.
- Moderate to severe decrease in menopausal hormone levels.

Menotype B's require more aggressive therapy than menotype A's, but with the correct natural protocol, they find significant improvement. In cases where herbal and other natural supplements are not effective enough, natural progesterone (I mainly recommend the cream form) can provide extra hormonal support. The body will convert some of the progesterone into estrogen, raising the level of that hormone as well. Other over-the-counter hormones such as DHEA and pregnenelone may also be indicated based on lab tests.

Menotype-B women may also show signs of the beginnings of osteoporosis, but they are usually close to average or mildly below average with regard to bone density when compared with other women their own age. Natural progesterone may have some benefit in protecting against this condition, although research has yet to give us definite

SHE TRIED IT

Jackie was a 54-year-old sales rep who had been suffering from menopausal hot flashes, anxiety, mood swings, and a slight reduction in libido for the past five years. Her father had died from heart disease. Her bone density was normal for her age and her blood work showed elevated cholesterol levels. Jackie had not been physically active for many years and was 30 pounds overweight. Her family doctor had recommended Premarin, but Jackie refused to take it. After consulting with her, I prescribed a typical menotype-B program. It included a herbal menopause formula consisting of Black Cohosh, and other hormone balancing herbs. I also recommended she take a separate herbal extract of Oatstraw to help with her anxiety. Nutritional supplements included vitamin E, CoQ10, calcium, magnesium, and a multivitamin without iron. I also had her start walking three times weekly for 20 minutes. Her dietary changes were simple: Include more fresh fish in her diet and eat more vegetables with her meals. After three months on this menotype-B protocol, her menopausal symptoms improved over 80 percent and Jackie lost 10 pounds. I then had her decrease the refined sugars and simple carbohydrates in her diet and increase her intake of legumes. At this point I also added an extra 400 IU of natural vitamin E and salmon oil to her program for increased cardiovascular protection. Jackie has been on this program for over two years and has been able to decrease the dosage of the herbs without an increase in menopausal symptoms. Her weight has continued to improve over time, and Jackie has noticed that if she eats too many refined sugar products, her weight will increase.

proof. Bone-supportive formulas are often recommended for menotype B's, besides the usual whole host of bone nutrients such as calcium, magnesium, vitamin D, boron, and so on. Hormone testing shows mild to moderate relative declines in their hormones.

The natural protocol for menotype B's is quite different from that of A's and C's. Here is a sample program, but be sure to read the rest of the book to tailor an individual program that's right for you.

Menotype-B Sample Program

- whole foods diet
- Black Cohosh extract or a Menopausal Herbal Formula **or** homeopathic **or**
- natural progesterone cream and/or DHEA and Pregnenlone
- high-potency multivitamin (without iron)
- vitamin E (mixed)—400 IU
- bone formula
- regular exercise
- condition-specific supplements depending on what is going on with you (for example, ginseng for energy, St. John's Wort for depression, vitamin C for the immune system)

NOTE: Cardiovascular-specific supplements are recommended if risk factors are present. See Chapter 10.

SHE TRIED IT

Frances was a 48-year-old with severe hot flashes and terrible night sweats. Her last period was over 6 months ago, indicating, along with bloodwork, that she was in menopause. Her saliva test showed normal decreases in most of her hormones, but her progesterone level was very low. Frances's bone density was slightly below normal for her age. I had her start treatment with natural progesterone, ipriflavone (supplement for her bones), calcium, magnesium, vitamin D, and several other minerals included in a formula. I also recommended she work with a trainer to start a weight-lifting and cardiovascular program. Frances was not interested in altering her diet. After one month, Frances reported an increase in energy and fewer hot flashes. Her night sweats had improved slightly but were still a problem. I prescribed an additional 400 IU of vitamin E as well as the homeopathic remedy Lachesis. This worked well for Frances and greatly improved the quality of her life during this transitional time.

Menotype C

The protocol for menotype C is very straightforward. Simply put, this category is for menopausal women who, for one reason or another, require hormone replacement therapy. This accounts for approximately 30–35 percent of all menopausal women we see in our clinic. The real decision comes down to whether to use "natural" or "synthetic" hormones.

In general, it makes sense to use hormones that are identical to those you find in the human body (and not what you find in a horse), so I tend to favor "natural" or "bioidentical" hormones over synthetic ones.

Hormone replacement may be necessary in any of several situations. The most obvious is the surgical removal of the ovaries (oophorectomy). In these cases, hormone replacement is especially recommended if the surgery took place before the menopausal years began. Intense hot flashes or vaginal dryness that do not respond to natural treatments, such as herbal and homeopathic therapy, can also be a signal that you need hormone replacement, as can very strong symptoms such as extreme night sweats.

SHE TRIED IT

Anne, a 49-year-old housewife, had not been feeling well since entering into menopause 8 months ago. On the request of her doctor, she had a bone-density study (DEXA scan) done. The results showed that Anne had significant bone loss. A special urine test that measures markers of bone loss was also done. As expected, it was higher than normal. Other tests also revealed deficiencies in many hormones. Anne was put on an aggressive treatment that included natural estrogens, natural progesterone, testosterone, and DHEA. We also prescribed a host of supplements including a bone formula that included Ipriflavone, as well as calcium, magnesium, vitamin D, boron, and many other minerals. She began an exercise program consisting of daily walking and weight training three times a week. Over the next year repeat urine tests showed that she was not turning over and losing bone as rapidly as she was before. A follow-up bone-density test 18 months after beginning treatment showed no further bone loss. Anne continues on the program today, with the hope of increasing her bone mass.

Another strong indicator for hormone replacement is osteoporosis. Because bone density can decline rapidly when a woman enters menopause, it's very important to begin therapy quickly, especially when osteoporosis is already present. Aggressive hormonal replacement is recommended and should include estrogen, progesterone, testosterone, DHEA, and, in some cases, growth hormone.

Elevated cholesterol and lipids, as well as other cardiovascular risk factors, may improve with estrogen replacement (as they can with diet, exercise, and supplements), but postmenopausal women who already have coronary artery disease won't see their condition go away. There are, of course, other ways to reduce risk factors when it comes to heart disease. You can, for example, start a program of regular exercise, use some stress management, and quit smoking. You can also use natural therapies to modify other risk factors, such as elevated homocysteine and blood pressure. Obviously, hormone replacement is not the only solution to cardiovascular disease prevention.

SHE TRIED IT

Melinda, a 53-year-old secretary, came to our clinic after being on Premarin® for over 4 years, which was originally prescribed by her family doctor for severe hot flashes and night sweats. Although she no longer had hot flashes or night sweats, Melinda did not "feel right." She suffered from breast tenderness and depression, as well as poor circulation. Her hands and feet would get very cold, even in the summertime. Our assessment was that Melinda was "sensitive" to the Premarin®, which was also contributing to a sluggish thyroid (confirmed by her low basal body temperature readings). I converted her medications to natural estrogen and natural progesterone, and prescribed the homeopathic remedy Natrum Muriaticum for her sluggish thyroid and depression. In addition, Melinda went on a liver-cleansing program to detoxify her body from the years of synthetic hormone use. Within two weeks of starting the new program, Melinda experienced a lifting of her depression and energy. Over the next three months, her cold hands and feet improved but it was not until she began taking Ginkgo that they returned completely to normal.

With regard to hot flashes, hormones should do the trick when the proper dosage is prescribed. Other menopausal therapies, such as Black Cohosh, need not be used for this particular symptom when HRT is prescribed. That doesn't mean, however, that you should altogether stop using herbal and nutritional supplements, or natural therapies such as homeopathy and acupuncture. Just the opposite. They can help smooth out menopausal symptoms that the hormone replacement does not correct. Poor memory, for example, may require Ginkgo, and dry skin may require flaxseed or fish oil.

As with menotype B's, diet does not usually make a pronounced impact on menopausal symptoms of menotype C's, but, of course, a good diet optimizes vitality and decreases risk of other diseases. However, since women on this program require hormones, they should consume phytonutrients that assist the liver in hormone metabolism, so that toxic metabolites do not build up and initiate other problems such as breast cancer. More on that later.

Menotype-C Sample Program

- natural estrogen and natural progesterone cream and/or DHEA and Pregnenlone (and potentially other hormones as well)
- phytonutrients that assist hormone metabolism (such as D-glucarate, Indole 3 carbinol, Rosemary extract, Sulforaphane, Silymarin, greem tea)
- high-potency multivitamin (without iron)
- vitamin E (mixed)—400 IU
- bone formula
- condition-specific supplements depending on what is going on with you (such as ginseng for energy, St. John's Wort for depression, vitamin C for the immune system)
- whole foods diet
- regular exercise

NOTE: Cardiovascular-specific supplements are recommended if risk factors are present. See Chapter 10.

As I discuss in Chapter 9, there is flexibility among the menotype classifications. Depending on your symptoms and risk factors, you may in time switch menotypes. For example, a menotype A may, at some point, develop the need for a menotype B program, and a B may need the C protocol, and so on.

2

$\mathscr{U}$NDERSTANDING
THE TRANSITION

$\mathscr{W}$hen you enter menopause, you essentially experience a "shutting down" of your reproductive system, which creates hormonal change and infertility. That's the simple version, and we're so used to accepting it that we take it for granted. But why, in fact, does the process happen?

Each woman is born carrying approximately 6 million ovarian eggs. By the time she reaches puberty, the number has decreased to about 300,000, and has fallen to somewhere in the neighborhood of 2,000 to 10,000 by the start of menopause. Why? The follicles that bear the eggs are thought to atrophy over the years due to nature's genetic programming. As a result, ovulation decreases and finally stops altogether. When that process nears its end, the body makes hormonal adjustments to compensate, and we enter perimenopause.

During the time of perimenopause, ovulation is erratic. Women often begin having what are called *anovulatory* cycles, which means no egg is released but monthly menstrual flow still occurs (causing many women to believe, incorrectly, that they are ovulating).

It is important to know that although the ovaries also stop producing progesterone during these cycles, they continue to manufacture estrogen. In fact, estrogen levels don't actually decline until six months or a year before a woman is in menopause. Thus, your estrogen levels can become very high, relative to your progesterone levels.

The pituitary gland responds to this imbalance by releasing FSH (follicle-stimulating hormone) and LH (luteinizing hormone) in an attempt to stimulate the ovaries to release more eggs and progesterone. Since the ovaries are no longer sensitive to stimulation from these hormones, estrogen levels finally begin to decline, and progesterone levels fall even further.

GETTING TO KNOW YOUR MENSTRUAL CYCLE

Acquiring an understanding of how your menstrual cycle has worked throughout your life will help provide you with a better understanding of what is happening during perimenopause and menopause.

You're familiar with the fact that the "normal" menstrual cycle is composed of 28 days. In reality, many women don't have a 28-day cycle, but for our purposes, let's assume that "magic" number.

Days 1–5, when menstruation occurs, are known as the menstrual phase. This event happens in response to declining levels of estrogen and progesterone, and is important because your uterus needs to shed its lining (endometrium) so that it does not grow too thick (and potentially turn cancerous).

On days 6–14, bleeding stops and the follicular phase begins. Now the endometrium again thickens, preparing the uterus for implantation. At the beginning of this phase, follicle-stimulating hormone (FSH) increases and helps a developing follicle reach maturity. Estrogen levels then rise, which leads to the suppression of FSH, and the pituitary gland releases LH to promote ovulation.

The third and final phase is the secretory phase, which comprises days 15–28. Now the follicle ruptures and the egg is released so that it can travel through the fallopian tube to the uterus. The ruptured follicle releases large amounts of progesterone, which stimulates growth of the endometrial lining to prepare for possible implantation and pregnancy. If there is no implantation, then progesterone levels drop and the menstrual cycle begins again.

28-DAY MENSTRUAL CYCLE
BEFORE MENOPAUSE

Days 1-5

- Bleeding begins.

- The decline of estrogen and progesterone hormones signals uterus that pregnancy has not occurred.

- Follicle-stimulating hormone (FSH) rises prior to ovulation, causins follicles in the ovaries to grow.

Days 6-14

- Estrogen rises.

- FSH begins to fall.

- The endometrial lining of the uterus thickens, in preparation for possible implantation of the fertilized egg.

Day 14

- Estrogen helps stimulate a large and sudden release of luteinizing hormone (LH), a hormone secreted to cause ovulation.

- LH surge causes follicle to rupture, and the egg is expelled into the fallopian tube.

Days 14-28

- Immediately after ovulation, the follicle bursts and becomes a *corpus luteum*.

- The *corpus luteum* begins secreting large amounts of progesterone.

- If the egg is not fertilized, the *corpus luteum* continues to release hormones until it runs out of them.

- The process begins again.

CRAZY MENSTRUAL PERIODS

Irregular vaginal bleeding occurs as a result of all these changes. Menstruation comes at unpredictable intervals, and often the time between menses shortens. For some women, the flow becomes light and brief. Others have extended bouts of very heavy bleeding. Other variations can occur, of course, depending on the woman.

It is important that women who have irregular bleeding during premenopause or postmenopause consult with a doctor. They'll want to make sure their symptoms are due to hormonal changes associated with the transition and not some other condition (such as endometrial cancer, polyps, fibroids, or other abnormalities). They'll also want to make certain they're not becoming anemic. Some of my patients had such heavy flow that they needed to be hospitalized to bring it under control.

WHAT IS UNUSUAL BLEEDING?

Irregular or abnormal bleeding refers to one or more of the following:

- intervals of 21 days or less
- seven days or more of bleeding
- heavy bleeding or very light (scanty) bleeding
- any other irregular patterns (for example, bleeding or spotting between cycles)

MORE ABOUT HORMONES

During the premenopausal years, the ovary is the chief producer of estrogen, specifically the type of estrogen known as estradiol. The ovaries produce far less estrogen after menopause. The main type of estrogen produced during this period is known as estrone, which is made by fat (adipose) tissue. That's why slender women produce less estrone than obese women and are more susceptible to menopausal symptoms. On the other hand, although obese women have less intense menopausal symptoms, they're at greater risk for breast and uterine cancer.

ADRENAL POWER

After the ovaries greatly reduce their production of estrogen and progesterone, the female body switches to its emergency backup system: the adrenal glands. Located on top of each kidney, the adrenal glands produce hormones, such as adrenaline and noradrenaline, that help your body deal with stress more effectively. A separate portion of the adrenal glands produces many other hormones.

Unlike your ovaries, the adrenal glands produce hormones all during your lifetime. When ovarian production of estrogen and progesterone (and other hormones) decreases in women during perimenopause, the adrenal glands pick up the slack. Specifically, they secrete the hormone pregnenelone, which is then used as a precursor to form other hormones such as DHEA, progesterone, androstenedione, estrogen, testosterone, and others. So your adrenal glands are important in maintaining production of your sex hormones.

We commonly find women (and men for that matter) who have had prolonged bouts of stress in their life suffering from deficiencies and imbalances of these adrenal hormones, along with others like cortisol (another stress hormone). This has the effect of leaving these women with more difficult and intense menopausal symptoms.

When we treat this adrenal "weakness," often referred to by practitioners as "adrenal fatigue or burnout," we find that many symptoms improve, including fatigue, depression, suppressed immune function, allergies, inflammatory conditions (for example, rheumatoid arthritis), low libido, and, to a lesser degree, hot flashes. Herbal supplements that are effective for strengthening the adrenals include the various Ginsengs, Licorice Root, Astragalus, and Ashwagandah (see more detail in Chapter 3). Nutritional supplements specific for the adrenals, which I recommend, can include vitamin C, vitamin B5, B6, zinc, and beta carotene. In more severe cases, supplementing with adrenal hormone precursors such as pregnenelone, DHEA, and, in some cases, cortisol helps. Of course, there is no replacement for good old "rest" and stress-reduction techniques.

THE BRIGHT SIDE OF CHOLESTEROL

You've probably read that cholesterol is a nasty substance, a major contributor to cardiovascular disease. Actually, you couldn't live without cholesterol. It not only allows cells to function properly, but it also serves as the precursor for all hormones. That's right, all of them! That's why sometimes I recommend underweight women with hormone imbalance symptoms (such as no menses or irregular menses) consume more cholesterol-containing foods to boost their hormone production.

MORE ABOUT HOT FLASHES

"For a minute or so I just sit there while sweat pours out of my face and chest pores. People who see me are always asking if I am all right, thinking I am having a heart attack or panic attack or something."

Menotype A: Hot flashes rare or nonexistent

Menotype B: Likely to occur

Menotype C: Frequent, including night sweats

Hot flashes are the most common symptom women in the United States experience during menopause: Approximately 75–85 percent of American women will have them. Hot flashes can occur months or years before your last period. In fact, they're not uncommon among women in their early 40's. Some women continue to have hot flashes ten years or more after menopause is over.

The characteristic hot flash (sometimes referred to by my patients as a hot flush or "power surge") begins in the head and face with a sudden sensation of warmth, followed by flushing of the skin. Next, the pulse goes up and the body temperature comes down as perspiration cools the skin, which is why some women may feel "chills" after a hot flash.

The symptoms can radiate down the neck or to other parts of the body. The flush is often followed by a large amount of perspiration in that area. The average hot flash is 2.7 minutes long. If the hot flash occurs during the night, it is called a "night sweat."

Researchers Need to Do More Work

You would think medical researchers would have pinpointed the exact cause of hot flashes by now, but alas, they haven't.

The most accepted theory at this point is that hot flashes are the result of a change in the body's thermostat, which is located in a section of the brain called the hypothalamus. The "set point" of a woman's thermostat may become lowered during perimenopause, causing a "heating up" reaction at relatively low temperatures.

You will often read in medical textbooks that hot flashes are the result of low estrogen levels, but that doesn't explain why prepubertal girls or women during menopause don't generally experience hot flashes, despite low levels of estrogen. So the explanation is probably more complex than "estrogen depletion."

It is known that the temperature-regulation area of the brain contains both estrogen and progesterone receptors. Many women have reported to me that natural progesterone works well to relieve their hot flashes. Thus, both estrogen and progesterone likely play a role in "modifying" or affecting your body's thermostat, although the mechanism is not well understood.

It is also thought that other neurotransmitters (brain chemicals) such as norepinephrine may be involved in causing hot flashes. And some researchers believe that brain opiates and endorphins get out of balance during the menopausal changes.

What to Do

Fortunately, even if we don't know why hot flashes happen, we do know a lot about how to reduce or stop them. Here are some things to try.

DON'T SMOKE. Women who smoke have more of a problem with hot flashes, so quitting may not only reduce your susceptibility to cancer, heart disease, and other smoking-related diseases, but may also help reduce menopausal symptoms as well.

EAT VEGETABLES. Vegetarians have fewer hot flashes. As I mentioned in the first chapter, studies have shown that Mayan and Japanese women have fewer problems with hot flashes, which is most likely the result of diet (high in plant foods containing phytoestrogens), exercise, and cultural views toward menopause.

STAY COOL. Obviously it makes sense to avoid hot environments. With some humor, many women tell me they fight over the bed sheets at night with their husband/partner as they throw off the covers while the husband pulls them back on. It's helpful to dress in layers so you can take layers off when hot.

KEEP YOUR DIET CALM. Spicy foods, alcohol, and caffeine products can also "aggravate" hot flashes for some women.

TRY HERBS. Herbs such as Black Cohosh and Vitex have been shown in several studies to be effective in reducing the frequency and intensity of hot flashes, and we find they work quite well.

GO HOMEOPATHIC. Specific homeopathic remedies such as Sepia, Pulsatilla, and Lachesis, to name a few, are relied upon by many women around the world to calm overwhelming hot flashes.

TRY VITAMINS. Even simple supplements such as vitamin E, usually in dosages of 800 IU or more, can be helpful.

ADD SOY. Soy, as a food and as a supplement, has become popular and has been proven in studies to reduce hot flashes.

USE NATURAL HORMONES. Women in the menotype-B category may require the use of natural progesterone by itself or in combination with the previous natural medicines listed. Natural estrogen works quite effectively for hot flashes and is often required in combination with progesterone and possibly other hormones for menotype C's.

ACCESS THE ALTERNATIVES. Don't forget that there are many other systems of medicine that can alleviate hot flashes. Acupuncture is one example that comes to mind which has gained much popularity in the past decade, and deservedly so.

WORK OUT. Exercise has also been shown to reduce the frequency of hot flashes.

Following the right menotype program should bring definite relief from your hot flashes—to the point at which they don't interfere with your daily activities or quality of life. Remember, hot flashes are not the symptoms of a disease and are a natural response. Thus, one cannot "cure" hot flashes but can manage them very effectively.

WHAT CAUSES THE OTHER SYMPTOMS

Insomnia

"I can't understand why I can't sleep. Stress in my life is at an all-time low," said Joyce. I then explained to her the connection of hormone changes with perimenopause and insomnia.

Menotype A: possible but not common (although may have been a problem long before perimenopause started)

Menotype B: common when perimenopause started

Menotype C: common and can be severe

Insomnia is a common problem during menopause. Some women have problems falling asleep while others wake up and then can't doze off again. Others sleep lightly but don't feel refreshed when they wake up because they haven't fallen into a "deep" slumber.

Researchers have looked into estrogen replacement for help with the problem, but results have been mixed. In my practice, I've found that looking at a broader hormonal picture can often provide better treatments.

Unbalanced levels of DHEA and cortisol can be at the root of insomnia. I frequently use a saliva hormone test that measures the levels of these hormones when treating women in menopause or any adult who has trouble falling asleep. Low melatonin may also be a problem, as can low levels of other hormones.

My female patients frequently tell me their doctors recommend a "sleeping medication" such as Valium for their insomnia. I don't care for this approach because of the dangers of addiction and overdosing and because, in my opinion, treating the cause of the insomnia makes far more sense than throwing drugs at the symptoms. That's why my patients rely on hormone-balancing supplements such as Black Cohosh, Vitex, or even natural hormones, depending on their menotype. The homeopathic remedies (see Chapter 7) can also work very well.

While addressing the underlying hormone imbalance, I may also recommend a temporary sleep aid. Three herbs that come immediately to mind are Passionflower, Hops, and Valerian Root. They help to calm the nervous system and promote relaxation and sleep. In addition, regular exercise and stress-reduction techniques, such as prayer before bedtime, can be quite helpful. For cases of insomnia that don't respond to other hormone therapies, melatonin sometimes works. Acupuncture may also aid in the relief of chronic insomnia.

Libido

"It's terrible. All my friends tell me what a hunk my husband is, yet I couldn't care less about having sex with him. It's the last thing on my mind, and he is getting quite upset about the whole situation," explained Sheila, a new patient of mine.

Menotype A: rare

Menotype B: common

Menotype C: can be a major problem

Many women report a decrease in libido or sex drive during menopause. There can be many factors related to a low libido, such as the health of one's relationship, stress and energy levels, and medical conditions such as depression. Hormone imbalances or deficiencies may also be at the root of the problem. If a woman tells me her libido was strong until she became perimenopausal and that there is no other explanation for the change she's experiencing, then I will strongly suspect a hormonal connection. Testing estrogen, progesterone, testosterone, and DHEA levels (which should be done anyway) can help shed light on major deficiencies or imbalances.

WHAT'S THAT "MALE HORMONE" (TESTOSTERONE) DOING THERE?

Mainly thought of as a male hormone, testosterone is also part of the female hormone family. The adrenal glands and ovaries produce testosterone. Production decreases as a woman ages, although it does not drop dramatically as estrogen and progesterone do during menopause. Testosterone use can be helpful for increasing libido, relieving vaginal dryness, maintaining bone density, increasing lean muscle mass, strengthening the immune system, and possibly protecting against heart disease. It has been shown that when used in combination with estrogen, it can help reduce hot flashes, night sweats, insomnia, and other symptoms of menopause that were unresponsive to estrogen therapy only. Too much testosterone, however, can lead to facial hair and other unwanted side effects, so the use of this hormone must be closely monitored.

Testosterone plays a role in the "sexual desire" of both men and women. However, I don't advocate that women with a low libido immediately start taking a testosterone replacement. Again, testing needs to be done to see if there is a significant deficiency. I have seen many patients whose libido improved nicely by balancing their estrogen and progesterone levels. Also, taking supplements of the hormone DHEA, which serves as a precursor hormone for testosterone, can be helpful.

Generally, the best approaches to this problem are those that have the least potential for harm. These include stress reduction, exercise, and natural supplements. Specific herbs such as Ginseng (especially Chinese or Panax Ginseng), Puncture Vine, Damiana, and Potency Wood can be quite helpful. (See Chapter 3.) In addition, homeopathic medicines, such as Sepia, work well to improve libido without the risk of toxicity that can occur with hormones. Acupuncture and Chinese herbal medicine can also be effective.

It's important to emphasize that libido and sexual arousal are strongly connected to the mind and emotions, and good communication is vitally important to having a fulfilling sex life with your partner.

The right words and actions from your partner may be all you need to improve your sexual response. Some of my patients need counseling with their partner to deal with issues that may be affecting their relationship and sex life. When these issues are worked out, the chances of a fulfilling sex life dramatically improve.

Headaches

As one patient told me, "The hot flashes aren't what bother me, it's those darn headaches. It feels like my temples are going to explode."

> Menotype A: rare (unless connected with a problem unrelated to menopause)
>
> Menotype B: common and moderately severe
>
> Menotype C: common and very severe

MIGRAINES. It's amazing how many women suffer from migraine headaches resulting from a hormone imbalance. This not only happens to women during menopause, but to women of all ages. Bringing the hormones back into equilibrium can provide great relief. Of course, common medications such as aspirin or Tylenol may take away the pain, but they don't treat the root of the problem. The same goes for common migraine pharmaceuticals such as Imitrex.

Migraine headaches often start after beginning hormone replacement therapy. Adjusting the dosages or abandoning synthetic hormones for a more natural approach is the quickest and surest way to resolve the problem. Sometimes low thyroid function can be the culprit.

Diet can also play a role in causing migraines, by way of food sensitivities or reactions to preservatives such as MSG or other food additives. On the other hand, the omega-3 fatty acids found in cold-water fish, such as salmon, and flaxseed can help prevent these debilitating headaches.

TENSION HEADACHES. Many women begin to suffer from tension headaches as they enter menopause. Hormonal changes, as well as the stresses of modern life, can result in tight muscles of the neck, back, and face. Tight muscles, in turn, may impair circulation and/or cause muscle spasms. Nutrients such as calcium and magnesium also help to relax the nerves and muscles. Stress-reduction techniques and tissue-specific therapies such as massage, acupuncture, and chiropractic can relieve and prevent tension headaches.

Fuzzy Memory and Concentration

"We have got to do something about my memory. I can't focus at work and I am even forgetting simple things like where I left my car keys."

Menotype A: less common

Menotype B: common

Menotype C: common and the changes can be severe

Many women in premenopause and menopause discover that their memory is beginning to fail them. Although a part of the problem may be related to age, memory loss seems to be more pronounced during the menopausal transition. Rapid reduction of estrogen and declining levels of other hormones may well play a role in "fuzzy memory" and declining concentration. Among women who have just given birth, we often hear the same kind of complaint, which is a powerful clue that hormones are involved.

Of course, estrogen and progesterone are not the only culprits. Prolonged elevation of the hormone cortisol is believed to be a major risk factor for both age-associated memory impairment and Alzheimer's disease. Low thyroid function, which I find to be quite common in women, can also be at the root of both poor memory and depression.

Circulation problems must also be considered, as must nutritional deficiencies of B12, B6, folic acid, and essential fatty acids. A blood-sugar imbalance can also lead to cloudy thinking, as the brain uses glucose, a simple sugar, as its preferred fuel source. Thus, if your blood sugar is constantly rising and falling, your brain cells are not getting a steady supply of energy to function properly. People with hypoglycemia and diabetes need to pay particular attention to eating a balanced diet, as well as eating at regular intervals.

Food sensitivities can also lead to a "foggy mind." Among these are sensitivity to cow's milk, wheat, sugar, soy, citrus fruit, peanuts, and chocolate. Sleep disturbances can also account for problems with memory and concentration ability.

Depression

"I know that depression has become a problem this past year. Everything seems to be getting dark, and all I want to do is sleep all the time. I never answer the phone."

Menotype A: rare

Menotype B: common and usually moderate

Menotype C: common and can be bad enough to interfere with daily activities

Studies are mixed as to whether depression is more common among women during menopause, and if hormone replacement therapy, particularly estrogen replacement, is beneficial in preventing or alleviating it. Biochemically, we know that estrogen helps maintain the neurotransmitter serotonin, which is important for "good mood." Other hormones, such as progesterone, DHEA, cortisol, thyroid hormone, and others, are also probably involved in balancing the brain's neurotransmitters. We also know that sometimes synthetic hormones can actually trigger depression. Fortunately, we usually reverse this situation by converting the patient to using more natural approaches.

Psychological factors that contribute to depression, such as emotional traumas or the stresses of life, can be treated with counseling, prayer, and natural remedies, especially homeopathic medicines. As with many conditions, many other factors can also be part of the picture, including nutritional deficiencies (for example, B vitamins, essential fatty acids, amino acids), lack of exercise, and the use of certain pharmaceutical medications.

I find that most cases of menopause-associated depression respond very well to nutritional, herbal, exercise, homeopathic, and counseling therapies. A recent study showed that St. John's Wort was very effective in relieving depression in women during menopause. Of course, hormone balancing often needs to be addressed for long-term success. Needless to say, I try as much as possible to avoid pharmaceutical antidepressants, such as Prozac, which have their own list of side effects and treat symptoms rather than causes.

Hair Loss and Hair Growth

"Look at my hair, it's falling out in clumps. The worst is when I shower in the morning and see a ball of hair in the drain."

Menotype A: rare but can happen

Menotype B: common and mild to moderate

Menotype C: common and moderate to severe

Changes in hormone levels can cause hair loss during both perimenopause and menopause. Androgens, such as testosterone, are thought to be responsible for the problem. Enzymes that convert precursor hormones to testosterone (and its metabolite DHT), which increase their activity during perimenopause, are also thought to be involved.

The adrenal precursor hormone androstenedione may also play a role in hair loss, as may a low or a hyper functioning thyroid gland, nutritional deficiencies (especially B vitamins, essential fatty acids, and silica), and poor digestive function (usually low stomach acid). Some women who are taking synthetic hormones complain they began losing their hair after they started taking the pharmaceuticals. This is particularly true of women on Premarin®.

Fortunately, the answer to this problem is usually simple. For the most part, hair loss stops after a few months of a woman's following her specific menotype program.

Acne and Other Skin Conditions

"I never had acne on my face since I was a teenager. It's embarrassing."

Menotype A: mild

Menotype B: mild to moderate changes

Menotype C: moderate to severe

THE HAIR YOU DON'T WANT

Hair *loss* isn't the only hair problem the "change-of-life" can bring. Hair *growth* on highly visible areas such as the cheeks, chin, upper lip, and on other parts of the body, including the abdomen, may occur during the menopausal transition and afterward. The medical term for this excessive hair growth is *hirsuitism*. Most medical textbooks will point to excess levels of testosterone as the culprit. The key is to focus on balancing estrogen and progesterone ratios, and sometimes adrenal hormones such as DHEA and cortisol. The testosterone imbalance will then automatically start to level out and thus lessen hair growth on these visible areas.

Acne is a very hormone-dependent condition for both males and females. It appears those with acne have greater activity of the enzyme 5-alpha reductase in the skin, which converts testosterone to a metabolite known as DHT (dihydrotestosterone). This leads to an increase in the production of keratin, a protein substance that forms the outer layer of the skin. The rapid growth of keratin, in turn, causes a blockage of the skin pores. As a result, acne lesions form in the hair follicle.

Increased testosterone production also causes an enlargement of the sebaceous glands and higher amounts of sebum (the waxy oil in your skin). As a result, whiteheads and blackheads form because some of the sebum cannot escape through the pores. These blockages also allow bacteria and yeast to overgrow on the skin and cause inflammation.

Interestingly, research has shown that the herb Saw Palmetto may have a blocking effect on the enzyme 5-alpha reductase, and may be one of the reasons herbalists have had success using this herb for the treatment of acne. Zinc, essential fatty acids, and herbs such as Vitex and Burdock Root can be quite helpful as well, due to their hormone-balancing effect. Some women require dietary changes and improved digestion to enjoy long-term success. Natural progesterone can also be helpful, especially when the acne occurs for only a week or two each month.

Many women experience acne rosacea, a chronic inflammatory skin disorder wherein the cheeks, forehead, and nose turn red. It occurs among adults who have a fair complexion and is more common in women. Again, there is a correlation between hormone imbalance and this condition. I have seen a number of women on synthetic hormones with rosacea whose skin dramatically improves after they switch to a more natural hormone-balancing, menotype protocol. The same can be said of psoriasis and other chronic skin conditions.

Urinary Problems

"Don't make me laugh. . . . I'll wet my pants!"

Menotype A: rare or not at all

Menotype B: mild

Menotype C: can be severe

Declining hormonal levels can produce atrophy (shrinkage) of the tissues of the bladder and urinary tract, making them less elastic and thinner and giving rise to frequent urinary tract infections. Also, a decline in estrogen and progesterone can lead to changes in the pH balance (increase in pH) of the vagina. This can create an environment that destroys friendly bacteria, such as *lactobacillus acidophilus*, which would otherwise help to prevent infections from yeast and unfriendly bacteria.

You can stop recurring bladder infections in their tracks through the use of cranberry juice or extract, vitamin C, and immune-enhancing herbs such as echinacea. Drinking more water and avoiding sugar, caffeine, and alcohol products is sometimes helpful as well. Urinating after sexual intercourse is also a good idea. And, of course, hormone-balancing approaches work to treat the underlying susceptibility. Estriol cream applied in the vagina can work quite well, as can the use of natural progesterone.

THE EMBARRASSING BLADDER PROBLEM

Some women experience urinary incontinence during menopause. That means dribbling occurs, or they lose urine when laughing, sneezing, or during exercise. Why? Estrogen and other hormones are responsible for some of the "tone" of the bladder muscles that control urination, playing a role in the circulation and nerve flow to the urethra (outlet of the bladder) and urinary tract.

For urinary incontinence, a woman can strengthen the muscles that control urination through special pelvic exercises called Kegel exercises. Also, specific homeopathic medicines such as Causticum and Sepia are well known to help incontinence related to menopause. Specific acupuncture treatments can also help alleviate this condition, and many women find that natural hormone replacement improves or totally eliminates incontinence. This includes applying estrogen cream in the vagina.

Not surprisingly, some women report experiencing urinary problems after starting synthetic hormones or using certain pharmaceutical medications. The obvious solution would be to convert to natural hormones or herbal/homeopathic therapy and to change medications.

Weight Gain

"Tell me you have something I can take for my weight. I have gained 30 pounds the last couple of years."

> Menotype A: common but usually slight weight gain
>
> Menotype B: common and moderate weight gain
>
> Menotype C: common and can be pronounced weight gain

Many women who have struggled with weight gain throughout their life find the problem becomes even more difficult as they enter perimenopause, especially after beginning synthetic hormone replacement. Most of the extra pounds are probably attributable to water retention and thyroid suppression.

Besides leaving you with a poor self-image, weight gain increases your risk of serious medical problems such as diabetes and cardiovascular disease.

Studies are mixed as to whether weight gain is the result of hormone changes associated with menopause or whether it is mainly due to lifestyle factors such as lack of exercise. But, of course, both exercise and dietary intervention are important in dealing with the problem.

Vaginal Dryness

"It's not that my sex drive is low, it's that it hurts too much because I am so dry."

Menotype A: rare

Menotype B: common and mild

Menotype C: common and moderate to severe

One of the most troublesome problems for women during menopause (and for years after menopause) is vaginal dryness and thinning. Decreased levels of estrogen and other hormones can lead to thinning and dryness of the vaginal walls and vulva. In addition, the glands that produce lubricating mucus may shrink, and the vaginal canal may decrease in size and lose elasticity. Thus, the space between the vagina opening and cervix decreases as well, making irritation, itching, and pain during or after intercourse more likely.

Although synthetic estrogen can be helpful for vaginal dryness, more natural therapies are preferable. For some women, herbs such as Black Cohosh and/or homeopathic remedies may be sufficient to alleviate symptoms, along with lubricant jelly. Vitamin E applied topically also works well. For more serious cases, as found with menotype C's, intravaginal estriol cream works very well. Testosterone cream can also help combat these same problems.

Fatigue

"I was checked for mono and chronic fatigue syndrome by a specialist, and nothing showed up. The fatigue seemed to come on when all these menopausal things started happening."

Menotype A: rare

Menotype B: common and mild to moderate

Menotype C: common and moderate to severe

Low energy or fatigue is one of the most common reasons people see a doctor. It is also a common symptom of menopause. There can be many reasons for fatigue, including anemia, stress, low thyroid function, nutritional deficiencies, underlying disease, poor digestion, toxicity, and many others. Of course, among women experiencing perimenopause, a hormonal imbalance is also highly suspect.

When a woman follows the correct menotype program, an increase in energy is one of the first things she'll notice. Also, sometimes simply getting more sleep and regular exercise go a long way to improving energy.

Arthritis

"I have gone from jogging to gardening. My joints just can't seem to handle running anymore."

Menotype A: common

Menotype B: common

Menotype C: common and progression accelerates during and after menopause

Osteoarthritis is the most common form of the more than 100 types of arthritis. It affects over 40 million Americans (most over the age of 45). It involves degeneration of the joints, specifically the cartilage, which acts as a cushion between adjoining bones. Symptoms include stiffness, pain, tissue swelling, and crepitus (creaking of joints).

The development of osteoarthritis takes many years. However, it is often around the time of menopause (45–50) that women begin to notice their knees or other joints feeling stiff in the morning. Although not well researched, I have found that women's symptoms improve when they follow their menotype program. Hormones may play a role because of their effect on circulation and the immune system. Many wonderful supplements can be used to combat this condition, including Glucosamine and Chondroitin sulfate, MSM, bromelain, omega-3 fatty acids, and others.

Rheumatoid arthritis is another common form of arthritis. It involves more inflammation of the tissues and joints. It is this form of arthritis that I find to be commonly worsened through the use of synthetic hormones. Conversely, proper use of natural progesterone and adrenal hormones like DHEA can go a long way in reducing the symptoms and progression of this disease. Supplements, like Moducare®, that reduce the autoimmune reaction may be helpful.

WHAT CAUSES THE OTHER HEALTH RISKS

Osteoporosis

Invariably, two important health risks need to be addressed when a woman in perimenopause sees her doctor. The first is osteoporosis.

Menotype A: rare

Menotype B: common and usually mild to moderate bone loss

Menotype C: common and can be severe

An estimated one in two women will develop osteoporosis in her lifetime. Your bones, as living tissue, are constantly producing new cells and discarding old ones, a process called bone turnover. The key to fighting osteoporosis is to keep that turnover in balance, that is, to get rid of old cells only as fast as you can manufacture replacements.

Hormones, especially estrogen, have a major effect on bone metabolism, so estrogen replacement remains the conventional mainstay for preventing postmenopausal osteoporosis. Due to lower levels of estrogen during menopause and postmenopause, a hormone known as parathyroid hormone (PTH) remains relatively high and causes bone resorption (breakdown). However, although the loss of bone density speeds up during menopause, the actual process begins many years before, possibly as far back as a woman's early 20's.

Keep in mind that estrogen replacement can help reduce bone loss, but it usually does not increase bone density. Other hormones also appear to be as important as estrogen in controlling bone loss, including progesterone, DHEA, calcitonin, growth hormone while excesses of cortisol and insulin contribute to bone loss.

Health habits play a major role in the progression of osteoporosis. Control of diet, exercise, smoking, and other factors are very important in the prevention and treatment of this disease.

Heart Disease

The other important health risk is heart disease.

Menotype A: common

Menotype B: common

Menotype C: common

A lot of media attention focuses on breast cancer and osteoporosis risk for women during menopause, which is good, but let's not forget about the number-one killer: heart disease. Research has shown that estrogen replacement therapy helps to reduce some of the risk factors associated with heart disease.

As you know, estrogen levels decrease in women during perimenopause and menopause. Estrogen replacement therapy has been shown to decrease total cholesterol levels (as well as other "bad" cholesterol markers such as LDL, lipoprotein A, apolipoprotein B), increase good HDL cholesterol, decrease homocysteine, improve the flexibility of arteries, and act as an antioxidant. However, whether it actually reduces a woman's risk of heart disease is controversial and an issue I will address in more depth in Chapter 10.

In any case, there are many natural approaches and supplements/herbs that achieve the same benefits as estrogen in reducing heart-disease risk factors and without exposing women to the side effects associated with estrogen replacement.

Lifestyle, of course, plays a major role in one's risk of heart disease.

SHARING AND KEEPING A JOURNAL

It is helpful for both you and your doctor to keep a journal or chart of the symptoms you have been experiencing. Symptoms can be used to help decipher what is going on inside your body. Also, by tracking what you are experiencing, you can see how different therapies (for your specific menotype) are helping or not helping you. Here is a chart you can photocopy and use to track your symptoms. Present it to your doctor on your visits to allow for a quick scan of what you're experiencing.

NOTE: Rate the intensity of your symptoms as: 0—don't have; 1—mild; 2—moderate; 3—severe. This is the same rating as your menotype quiz in Chapter 1. The difference is that you will track these symptoms on a daily basis.

MONTHLY SYMPTOM CHART

Your Menotype _____

Symptoms	Day 1	Day 2	Day 3 ...
hot flashes			
night sweats			
insomnia			
depression			
fatigue			
irregular bleeding			
irritability			
mood swings			
anxiety			
loss of memory and concentration			
vaginal dryness			
urinary problems (incontinence or urinary tract infections)			
skin changes			
headaches			
joint pain			
heart palpitations			
vertigo (sensation of room turning or spinning)			

Symptoms	Day 1	Day 2	Day 3 ...
joint pain			
bloating			
flatulence			
breast tenderness			
low sex drive			
acne			
increase in facial hair			
hair loss			
food cravings			
other _____			
other _____			
other _____			

Summary of medications and supplements being taken this month: _____

_____

_____

_____

I also recommend you keep a file that contains your medical records. This should include past medical tests and notes, your completed menotype quiz, this monthly symptom chart, and any future lab tests or reports (hormone analysis, bone density, bloodwork, and so on).

CHOOSING YOUR DOCTOR

How do you know which healthcare provider is right for you? It might be the same person you've been seeing for the last 20 years. Then again, it might not.

Here are some criteria people have found helpful as a guideline in choosing a doctor, and in particular, women looking for a holistic approach to menopause.

1. **The doctor should be trained as a primary healthcare provider.** Currently, the only doctors I know who are trained as primary healthcare providers (meaning they can legally diagnose and treat disease) are medical doctors, osteopathic doctors, chiropractors, naturopathic doctors, and acupuncturists. Ideally, licensed naturopathic doctors have the most comprehensive training in conventional and natural medicine. (See the Resources at the back of this book to find a naturopathic doctor in your area.)

2. **The doctor should have a good reputation.** Talk to others who have seen this practitioner and ask about their experiences. Getting a referral makes more sense than blindly going to see a doctor.

3. **Investigate the doctor's philosophy and approach to health and menopause.** Does the doctor have training and experience in holistic therapies? If so, what kind of training and experience? If he or she basically recommends that every menopausal woman routinely receive HRT, find another doctor.

4. **He or she should use the most advanced techniques in diagnosis and clinical testing.** For example, you would want to ask if the doctor uses salivary hormone testing.

5. **The doctor should be a good listener.** It is important that you feel heard and understood. I usually spend an hour or more with a new patient to get a full history and to listen to the patient and her concerns.

6. **The doctor should be willing to make referrals.** No doctor is an expert in everything. A good holistic doctor will refer to a specialist when it is in the best interest of the patient to get better. Ask your doctor if he or she networks with other doctors and natural healthcare practitioners.

BEING GOOD TO YOURSELF

Remember, major hormonal and metabolic shifts occur during menopause. Your body needs adequate rest. The more you can relax, the easier the transition will be for you. Your stress glands (adrenals) need to be working optimally to make up for the shutting down of your ovaries. How about a few extra massages while this is going on? Many of my patients tell me they would love to get some massages to relax and get the kinks out of their muscles. Those who do are pleased with how they feel. You're worth it! So go ahead and schedule some massages or other stress-reducing techniques.

SHE TRIED IT

Sally, an enthusiastic banker, had been handling perimenopause pretty well with the menotype-B program, focusing on the herbal and nutritional supplements I had recommended. Sally had one problem, though, and that was a lagging libido. When asked if there were any emotional or psychological reasons why her sexual desire had decreased, she could not think of any, and she had no problems with pain during intercourse, which can happen during menopause due to thinning and drying of the vagina and clitoris. Further testing showed that her DHEA levels were getting quite low and that her testosterone was borderline low. Her libido started to increase after four weeks on DHEA supplementation, and by eight weeks she felt "like a teenager" again.

3

$\mathcal{N}$ATURE'S TOP HERBAL HORMONE BALANCERS

$\mathcal{A}$fter you work out your menotype and the particular regimen that's exactly right for you, you'll use a combination of herbs, food, exercise, and lifestyle "ingredients" that are uniquely suited to you.

The herbs mentioned in this chapter are very important for menotype-A women and even more so for menotype B's, as herbal medicines can be the primary treatment for these types. Herbs do *not* replace the use of hormones as primary therapy for menotype-C women, but they are very important in treating specific menopausal symptoms.

CHINA:
OLD RECORD OF HERBAL HEALING

One of the oldest formal records of herbal healing is found in Chinese lore. In 2735 B.C., Emperor Shen Nung wrote the first Chinese pharmacopoeia, *Pen Tsao Ching (The Classic of Herbs)*. Shen Nung is said to have self-tested hundreds of these herbs and compounds.

The first major Chinese medical work translated into Western languages was *Pen Tsao Kang Mu (The Catalogue of Medicinal Herbs)*. Written by Li-Shih-Chen during the late sixteenth century, this 52-volume work listed 12,000 prescriptions, and analyzed 1,074 plant substances and 354 mineral substances.

TEST OF TIME VERSUS TEST IN TUBE

Science is finally catching up with tradition. Today, researchers use sophisticated tools to determine an herb's identity and purity, as well as the amount of its active ingredient. Double-blind, placebo-controlled studies have confirmed the benefit of several herbs, including Black Cohosh *(Cimicifuga racemosa)*, Licorice Root *(Glycyrrhiza glabra)*, Ginseng *(Panax ginseng, Eleutherococcus senticosus, P. quinquefolius)*, Red Clover *(Trifolium pratense)*, St. John's Wort *(Hypericum perforatum)*, and Kava Root *(Piper methysticum)*.

We have certainly learned a great deal about herbal medicine through clinical trials, meta-analyses, and tools such as microscopes and chromatographic "fingerprinting." However, folk traditions were recommending these herbs for millennia before scientists studied them. In fact, medicinal plants have been found near Stone-Age sites, estimated to be about 12,000 years old.

HERBS IN EGYPT AND INDIA

Well before the birth of Christ, the peoples of China and India exchanged medical information. Ancient Indian medicine is called *ayurveda,* derived from two Sanskrit words: *ayur,* meaning "life," and *veda,* meaning "knowledge." Much of *ayurveda* comes from the oldest of India's four books of classic wisdom, the 4,500-year-old *Rig Veda*. This work includes extensive descriptions of plant medicines, using 67 herbs, among them Ginger, Cinnamon, and Senna.

Two millennia before the birth of Christ, as many as 2,000 herbal doctors were practicing in Egypt, according to the ancient *Ebers Papyrus*. This record traces over 1,000 years of ancient medicine and lists 876 herbal formulas made from more than 500 plants. Some of the recommendations have stood the test of time. For example, the Egyptians believed that garlic and onion strengthened the body and prevented disease. Modern research has confirmed the therapeutic value of garlic and onion.

GREECE AND ROME:
PLANT REMEDIES THRIVED

The Greeks and Romans also relied on herbal medicine. Greek philosopher Aristotle kept a garden of more than 300 plants he believed had medicinal value. Pedanius Dioscorides, also a Greek, as well as a physician with the emperor Nero's Roman legions, published his *De Materia Medica (On Medicines)* in 78 A.D. This work, which listed 600 medicinal plants, was used as a standard medical reference for 1,500 years. Dioscorides is considered the first true medical botanist.

The spread of herbal medicine throughout Europe is attributed to the spread of the Roman Empire. Roman armies took herbs with them on their travels, planting them along the way both inadvertently and by design.

CHRISTIANS:
CONTINUING THE TRADITION

The Christians picked up where the Romans left off. Benedictine and Cistercian monasteries were centers of herbal activity in the Dark Ages. The monks preserved ancient texts of herbal wisdom, and collected and cultivated as many plants as they could find.

The Benedictines also adopted the Arab practice of combining herbs with alcohol. They mixed digestion-enhancing herbs with wine and produced the forerunners of modern liqueurs.

The Bible itself makes reference to several herbs, among them Flax, Cinnamon, Cumin, Hyssop, Myrrh, Thistle, and Wormwood.

RENAISSANCE EUROPE:
FORMAL AND KITCHEN HERB GARDENS

In the capitals of Renaissance Europe, herbs became the focal point of elaborate, formal, ornamental gardens. Herbs also grew in abundance in the kitchen gardens of manors and smaller homes.

Flora Thompson, author of *Lark Rise,* in writing about village life in the 1880s, described how village women kept medicinal herb corners in their cottage gardens, with Horehound, Peppermint, Pennyroyal, Tansy, Balm, and Rue.

NATIVE AMERICANS: SHARING HERBAL WISDOM WITH COLONISTS

Native Americans found a use for almost every plant native to their land. When explorers and colonists came to the New World, many of the herbs they brought with them didn't grow well on North American soil. Furthermore, they were impressed by Native Americans' strong health, physical stamina, and good teeth.

The Native Americans were generous with their herbal wisdom, introducing the white settlers to healing herbs such as Black and Blue Cohosh, Echinacea, Cascara Sagrada, Goldenseal, Oregon Grape, Slippery Elm, and Witch Hazel.

BRITISH HERBALISTS

Three of the most prominent English herbalists were John Gerard, Nicholas Culpeper, and John Wesley. Gerard (1545–1612), who served as apothecary (that is, pharmacist) to King James I, published *Gerard's Herbal* in 1597. Culpeper (1616–1654) doctored in a London slum, seeing patients in his apothecary shop and often refusing to accept a fee. He recommended "cheap but wholesome Medicines . . . not sending them to the East Indies for Drugs, when they may fetch better out of their own Gardens." Culpeper published the *Complete Herbal and English Physician* in 1652, which has been in print in more than 100 editions ever since.

Although he made an enormous contribution to herbal medicine, Culpeper was also prone to exaggeration: He promoted dozens of herbs as cure-alls and linked herbs to astrology. Unfortunately, these beliefs made Culpeper—and herbalism—an easy target for ridicule.

Methodist preacher John Wesley (1703–1791) sold his book *Primitive Physic, or An Easy and Natural Way of Curing Most Diseases* (published in 1747) for pennies to people who couldn't afford professional medical help. Wesley espoused simple and effective remedies, as well as basic rules of preventive medicine.

TRADITIONAL HEALER VS. "PROFESSIONAL" PHYSICIAN

Roman physician Galen (first century A.D.) is considered the forefather of modern medicine. He classified the four humors (elemental body fluids) as blood, bile, phlegm, and choler. Humors were the basis of the teachings of the Hippocratic school.

Galen established the distinction between professional doctor and traditional healer. His system of medicine was so complex that only well-educated people could understand it.

Galen's system dominated European medical theory for 1,500 years. During that time, "professional" physicians tried to speed up healing with bloodletting, purging, and administering exotic—sometimes even toxic—medicines. This was in direct opposition to the traditional healer's reliance on herbs and nature's curative powers.

Many people lost faith in Galenic medicine during the Black Plague of 1348 A.D. Almost one-third of Europe's population died, and professional medicine was helpless to stop it. When syphilis emerged 150 years later, professional physicians used mercury—a highly poisonous substance—to treat it. At the same time, the spread of this disease revived interest in herbal intervention.

Samuel Thomson (1760–1843), early America's leading herbalist, loathed the professional physicians of his time, with their use of leeches and poisons. In 1839, he boasted three million followers, including Dr. John Kellogg of Battle Creek, Michigan, developer of the corn flake (one of our country's first commercial health food).

TAKE THESE AND CALL ME IN THE MORNING, MR. PRESIDENT

During the colonial era, most physicians relied on bloodletting, laxatives, and mercury to cure illnesses. Unfortunately, many of their patients paid the price. George Washington was one victim of such "professional" medical care. In 1799, he came down with chills, fever, and a sore throat. Rest, hot liquids, and herbal antibiotics—such as echinacea, garlic, and onion—would have probably cleared it up. However, his physicians took four pints of blood out of him, leaving him weak and anemic, and administered mercury and laxatives. Our first president was dead within 24 hours.

WHOLE HERBS VS. ISOLATED COMPOUNDS

Traditionally, people used whole herbs to treat illness and support health. Today, researchers have isolated the so-called "active ingredients" of many herbs, which are often recommended to address specific health concerns. This practice may make it easier to comply with Food & Drug Administration (FDA) regulations, but it is by no means the sole reason for an herb's overall medicinal impact.

All herbs contain a variety of compounds. Although one of these compounds may be primarily responsible for an herb's medicinal effect, some of the other ingredients can enhance its benefit, while still others may protect against possible side effects.

Consider Chinese Ginseng. Some researchers are narrowing their focus on Ginseng's antioxidant and cholesterol-lowering benefits. Yet Ginseng also has the ability to fight fatigue, improve blood-sugar balance, improve liver health, and protect against radiation. Ginseng also has several known active ingredients such as ginsenosides, which increase energy and stimulate nervous system and brain activity; as well as polyacetylenes and polysaccharides, which activate the immune system and possess anti-cancer activity. Yet, other compounds, which have not been identified, probably also contribute to its versatile effects.

HERBAL FORMULAS FOR SYNERGISTIC IMPACT

Today's herb manufacturers often combine a number of herbs in a single product.

While one herb may provide a particular action, other herbs in the formula enhance it or protect against its possible side effects. An herbal formula can address a full range of symptoms, whereas a single herb may be more limited. Consider the following herbs:

- **Black Cohosh** is particularly effective at relieving hot flashes and menopausal depression.
- **Chasteberry** alters secretions of luteinizing hormone (LH) and follicle-stimulating hormones (FSH) and is excellent for hot flashes.
- **Wild Yam Root** may help balance estrogen and progesterone levels in the body, and reduce breast tenderness and uterine cramping.
- **Licorice Root** supports adrenal gland function. The adrenal glands continue to produce estrogen and progesterone after the ovaries cease to function.
- **Hops** are used as a nerve tonic and mild sedative. They are also recommended for upset stomach and insomnia.

Single herbs such as Black Cohosh can be used alone to treat menopause. However, by combining these herbs into a single formula, you can treat the gamut of menopausal symptoms. Each herb has a different action on the body, so a synergistic combination can treat more symptoms. A blend of indicated herbs maximizes the chances of success.

TRADITION VS. SCIENCE

Specific uses for specific herbs have been surprisingly consistent through the centuries. The health-promoting properties of plants, first touted in folklore, are now supported by scientific evidence, and modern researchers are finding out how they work.

As science grants a new legitimacy to the traditional uses of plants, herbs are reclaiming their rightful place in natural healthcare. They are emerging as the medicine of the future as well as the past: a safe, effective approach to healing. They work for my family and me, and they can work for you.

IS THERE ONLY ONE PREFERRED FORM
OF HERBAL MEDICINE?

There is no one universally preferred form of herbal medicine. Many people prefer using the capsule form, as it is potent, convenient to use, and has no taste. Other people don't like to swallow capsules or tablets, and they often prefer to use a tea, tincture, or fluid. Some herbs, of course, are excellent foods. Take garlic and onion, for example, which can benefit the cardiovascular and immune system even when used as spices in meals.

In some cases, using standardized extracts produces better results. For example, to help with memory and circulation, you're far better off using a standardized form of Ginkgo (usually capsule) than the tea form. Also, when successful scientific studies have specifically tested use of a standardized extract, it makes sense to follow their protocol. For example, several studies have found St. John's Wort, at a specific dosage (900 mg) of a 0.3% hypericin extract, helps relieve depression. Since you know that works, why would you use another form or dosage of the herb?

Cost is another factor. It's a whole lot cheaper to buy some Ginger Root at the store and make your own tea than to buy a commercial version in tea bags or capsules.

Here are some general rules of thumb:

- Decoctions and infusions are the most affordable forms of plant medicines, especially if you grow the herbs yourself.

- Tinctures and fluid extracts are more potent than herbal teas.

- Capsules and tablets, which are standardized herbal extracts, generally offer the most consistency.

MENOPAUSE-SPECIFIC HERBS

Black Cohosh (Cimicifuga racemosa)

Black Cohosh is a perennial herb native to North America. It has been popular among Native Americans, early North American colonists, Chinese and Japanese traditional doctors, midwives, and modern-day herbalists. Black Cohosh rhizome (underground plant stem) was included in the *United States Pharmacopeia* from 1820 until 1936. Today, the German Commission E (Germany's equivalent of the Food & Drug Administration) approves Black Cohosh for menopausal symptoms, painful menstruation, and premenstrual discomfort.

APPLICATIONS. Black Cohosh has been shown to relieve menopause-related hot flashes, depression, and vaginal dryness. It is also reported to relax muscles, decrease pain, and soothe the nerves.

HOW IT WORKS. Researchers disagree on how exactly Black Cohosh relieves menopausal symptoms. There is some literature that supports the idea that levels of LH (lutenizing hormone) are lowered with Black Cohosh supplementation. During menopause, estrogen and progesterone levels drop, while the pituitary gland increases levels of LH. The rise in LH is believed to be one of the reasons why menopausal symptoms occur. So the inhibition of LH release by the pituitary gland is why menopausal symptoms are relieved with Black Cohosh. Some researchers feel that estrogen-balancing chemicals, known as phytoestrogens, in Black Cohosh may act to relieve menopausal symptoms as well.

CLINICAL STUDIES. Several studies have looked at Black Cohosh and its effect on menopausal women. As with many herbs, most of the research has been done in Europe (Germany).

A study by Stolze of 131 doctors and 629 female patients revealed that a standardized extract of Black Cohosh alleviated menopausal symptoms in over 80 percent of the patients within six to eight weeks. Many women noticed improvement within four weeks of use. Symptoms that improved included hot flashes, headaches, vertigo, heart palpitations, nervousness, ringing in the ears, anxiety, insomnia, and depression.

In another study, 80 menopausal women were given either Black Cohosh, synthetic estrogen, or a placebo for 12 weeks. Those who took the Black Cohosh had the best results in relieving menopausal symptoms including reduced anxiety and decreased hot flashes. This study is quite powerful as it provides some evidence of the effectiveness of Black Cohosh when put head to head with estrogen replacement.

DECOCTIONS, INFUSIONS, CAPSULES, AND OTHER FORMS OF HERBAL MEDICINE

Herbs come in many different forms, among them decoctions, infusions, tinctures, fluid extracts, and standardized extracts.

- **Decoctions** are used to allow the ingestion of harder plant parts such as the bark, seeds, and root (for example, raw ginger root). You make a decoction by heating the herb (one tablespoon of dry herb or three tablespoons of fresh herb) in water until it boils and letting it simmer (cover with a lid) for 15 to 25 minutes. Then let it sit for 10 minutes, strain, and serve.

- **Infusions** are teas made from the softer parts of herbs, such as leaves and flowers. Peppermint Leaf is a classic example. Commercial preparations of tea bags are available, or you can use dry or fresh herbs. For tea bags, add one bag to a cup of boiled water and let sit for 10 to 15 minutes. For dry or fresh herbs, bring one cup of water to a boil in a kettle (then turn off heat) and add one tablespoon of dry herb or three tablespoons of fresh herb to the water. Cover with a lid and let sit for 10 to 15 minutes. Strain and serve.

- **Capsules** contain the dry powder of the herb. They are popular because of their convenience: easy to take, as there is no taste involved, and easy to store in containers. Most of my patients prefer this form.

- **Tinctures** are herbs soaked in a solvent, typically alcohol and water, for a specific amount of time. Typically, tinctures are considered less potent than fluid extracts or standardized extracts. Tincture concentration is usually 1:5 or 1:10, which means that one part of herbal material is used with five or ten parts of the solvent.

- **Fluid extracts** are considered more potent than tinctures, infusions, or decoctions. The concentration of a fluid extract is usually 1:1, which means one part herbal material is used with one part solvent.

- **Solid extract.** By removing all fluid, a solid extract is created that can either be put into a capsule or tablet.

- **Standardized extracts.** Utilizing scientific techniques, an isolated compound within the plant, known to cause a therapeutic effect, is targeted. Standardization insures that each capsule will show this same amount of therapeutic activity. While the whole herb is used, the same level of isolated active component is maintained. Tinctures can be standardized as well.

Researchers have also studied women who were making a transition from hormones to Black Cohosh. One such study found 28 out of 50 women were able to make the switch to Black Cohosh without taking additional hormones.

RECOMMENDED DOSES. I recommend a Black Cohosh extract standardized to 2.5% triterpene glycosides. The typical dosage used in studies for the relief of menopausal symptoms was 80 mg in tablet form (one can use capsule) or 80 drops of tincture. Most women notice improvement within four weeks of starting supplementation. For severe menopausal symptoms or for women who do not see improvement at 80 mg, I recommend using 160 mg daily. In time, usually after six months or longer, one may be able to reduce the daily dosage to 80 mg.

POTENTIAL SIDE EFFECTS. Side effects are uncommon with Black Cohosh. As with many herbs, digestive upset occurs in a small percentage of users, but you can eliminate this side effect by taking Black Cohosh with food. Clinical studies involving more than 1,700 patients over a three- to six-month period showed excellent tolerance of Black Cohosh. Much higher dosages than I recommend may result in headaches and dizziness. Black Cohosh should be avoided during pregnancy and while breastfeeding.

I am often asked if women with a history of breast or uterine cancer can safely use Black Cohosh. Researchers have looked at this question, and their conclusions are reassuring. One study showed that breast cancer cells whose growth is dependent on estrogen are not stimulated by Black Cohosh. As a matter of fact, just the opposite: Black Cohosh helped to stop cancer cells from proliferating. The main action of Black Cohosh is that it alters the levels of hormone production in the body instead of actually supplying hormones. The German Commission E states that Black Cohosh appears to be safe in women with a history of breast cancer.

Some sources state that Black Cohosh should not be used for more than six months. I disagree with this. Although long-term use has not been well studied, I have found no problems among my patients and cannot see why there would be any. Certainly it is safer than hormone use.

Vitex (Vitex agnus-castus) *or Chasteberry*

DESCRIPTION.   Vitex, also commonly referred to as Chasteberry, is a shrub that grows in the Mediterranean and Central Asia. After pollination, a dark-brown fruit develops, which is about the size of a peppercorn.

Vitex has long been used to treat female maladies. In the fourth century B.C., Hippocrates, considered the father of modern medicine, recommended Vitex for uncontrolled bleeding after childbirth. In the first century A.D., Pliny, the Greek natural historian, wrote that "The trees furnish medicines that promote urine and menstruation." Gerard, European herbalist in the sixteenth century, recommended chasteberry as a "female" herb. He claimed it would relieve the pain and inflammation of the uterus.

Although Black Cohosh is the most specific herb for menopause, Vitex is also helpful and has more applications for women's overall health.

APPLICATIONS.   Vitex is used to treat menstrual complaints, premenstrual syndrome (PMS), infertility, fibroids, ovarian cysts, endometriosis, acne, menopause, and breast tenderness.

HOW IT WORKS.   By changing the volume of secretions of follicle-stimulating hormones (FSH) and luteinizing hormones (LH), vitex may relieve menopausal symptoms, especially hot flashes. Vitex may raise progesterone levels. Low levels of progesterone are implicated in premenopausal and menopausal symptoms. A "luteal phase defect" occurs when estrogen controls the second half of the menstrual cycle, too, because there's not enough progesterone. This makes Vitex effective for irregular and heavy menstrual cycles that occur during perimenopause.

Physicians in Europe commonly recommend Vitex for the treatment of hot flashes. Although I have not seen any literature as to how Vitex specifically relieves hot flashes, altering the FSH and LH probably has a lot to do with its effectiveness.

CLINICAL STUDY.   Widely used by physicians in Europe, Vitex has been studied for its benefit of relieving hot flashes. Some research does show, however, that it can successfully treat PMS. Well-known herbalist

Christopher Hobbs comments in his book *Vitex: The Women's Herb,* "Vitex and preparations containing the herb are the most widely-used natural medicine in Europe for helping to relieve unpleasant symptoms that may occur before, during, and after menopause, being recommended by herbalists and physicians alike."

RECOMMENDED DOSES. Clinical studies generally used a daily dosage equivalent to 30 mg to 40 mg of the dried fruit. In terms of commercial products, I generally recommend a standardized extract containing 0.6% aucubin at a dosage of 160 to 240 mg daily. It can also be taken in tincture form at a dosage of 40 drops, one to three times daily. For patients going through menopause, I typically recommend Vitex be used with other herbs listed in this chapter.

POTENTIAL SIDE EFFECTS. Occasionally, Vitex may lead to skin rashes and digestive upset. It is not recommended for pregnant women, nursing mothers (unless they're taking it under a doctor's guidance), or women who are taking drugs that block dopamine receptors, such as haloperidol and women on birth control pill.

Wild Yam Root (Dioscorea villosa)

Wild Yam Root is a twining perennial vine with small, greenish-yellow flowers. It is native to the southern United States and Canada. However, it is now widely cultivated in tropical, subtropical, and temperate regions throughout the world.

APPLICATIONS. Herbalists have traditionally used Wild Yam to treat menopause, menstrual disorders, miscarriage, infertility, and endometriosis.

HOW IT WORKS. Wild Yam does not supply progesterone. It does contain a steroidal saponin known as diosgenin. Diosgenin in a laboratory setting (not in the body) acts as the precursor (basic ingredient) for the production of estrogen, progesterone, and pregnenolone.

Wild Yam Root may help balance estrogen and progesterone levels in the body. It has also been shown to mildly lower triglycerides (fats) and raise HDL ("good") cholesterol in the blood.

THE WILD YAM SCAM

Wild Yam *(Dioscorea villosa)* is a member of the vast *Dioscorea* family, which includes the common potato. *Dioscorea* foods are named after Dioscorides, the renowned first-century Greek physician. His writings on medicinal herbs were the standard for more than a millennium.

Wild Yam contains a compound called diosgenin. Some advertisements claim that the body converts the diosgenin content of Wild Yams into hormones such as pregnenolone and progesterone. This is untrue; the conversion of diosgenin to hormones needs to be done in a lab. Most of the confusion comes out of creams marketed as Wild Yam extract, which give the illusion that it is a natural progesterone cream. If you are looking for a cream that contains natural progesterone, make sure to ask if it is a reputable brand and actually contains progesterone before buying it.

I do not find Wild Yam to be effective by itself in relieving menopausal symptoms, but do find it a great synergistic herb in menopausal formulas.

RECOMMENDED DOSES. In a formula, I recommend 75 to 300 mg of a 10:1 concentrated extract to be taken two to four times daily. If taken by itself, the dosage is 30 to 60 drops or 500 mg of a nonstandardized capsule twice daily.

POTENTIAL SIDE EFFECTS. Wild Yam is nontoxic, although large doses may cause nausea.

Licorice Root (Glycyrrhiza glabra)

Licorice Root is yellowish-brown in color. The plant is a perennial with bluish to pale violet blossoms.

Licorice Root is one of the most extensively used and scientifically researched botanical remedies. It has been utilized therapeutically since at least 500 B.C. and has been cultivated in Europe since the sixteenth century. Licorice *(Glycyrrhiza uralensis)* has also been one of the most popular compounds in Chinese medicine formulas for over 3,000 years.

APPLICATIONS. Licorice Root is used to treat symptoms of menopause and premenstrual syndrome (PMS), peptic ulcers, asthma, and canker sores. It is also used to support adrenal gland function, especially after the use of cortisone.

HOW IT WORKS. Licorice contains isoflavones that have estrogen and progesterone balancing compounds. These compounds appear to decrease estrogen levels in women when they're too high, and increase the levels when they're too low.

Licorice also supports adrenal gland function. The adrenal glands continue to produce estrogen and progesterone after the ovaries cease to function, although at decreased levels. Glycyrrhizin is an important constituent that improves the effects of cortisol in the body (powerful anti-inflammatory and anti-allergy effects) without the side effects of pharmaceutical versions such as prednisone. It also slows down the formation of prostaglandins, which cause inflammation.

RECOMMENDED DOSES. Licorice Root is best used in small dosages in menopausal formulas. I commonly recommend a capsule containing 75 mg, to be taken two to four times daily. The tincture dosage is 10 to 15 drops two to three times daily.

POTENTIAL SIDE EFFECTS. Chronic use of regular Licorice Root may trigger water retention, high blood pressure, and excessive loss of potassium. These effects are reversible. However, adverse effects are rarely noted at intake levels below 3,000 mg daily of the powdered extract or 100 mg of glycyrrhizin per day. I would recommend a low-sodium, high-potassium diet if you're concerned about elevated blood pressure.

In addition, Licorice Root is not recommended for individuals with a history of high blood pressure or kidney failure, or those who use digitalis medications.

Hops (Humulus lupulus)

Hops come from a vine with cone-like fruiting bodies.

LABEL READING

When choosing an herbal product, it is critical to read the label closely. A label for an herbal product should provide the following information:

- Product name
- Identity statement
- Lot number
- Expiration date
- Ingredient listing with amounts
- Other ingredients (if any)
- Directions/dosage
- Warnings (if any)
- Size (number of tablets/capsules)
- Manufacturer/distributor information

Here are some general questions you should ask yourself about the product(s) you are considering:

1. Are there instructions for use, as well as warnings or contraindications (what the product should not be used with)? The more complete the label is, the better chance it is a high-quality product.

2. Does the product have an intact, tamper-resistant seal? Remember, the tamper-resistant seal is there for a reason.

APPLICATIONS. Hops have been used traditionally as a nerve tonic and mild sedative. It has also been used to treat upset stomach and insomnia.

HOW IT WORKS. Hops are powerful phytoestrogens. According to herbalist Rosemary Gladstar, "Hops contain high concentrations of plant hormones that have estrogen-like effects on the female system." This phytoestrogen effect balances estrogen levels in the body. As a nerve tonic, Hops help calm the nerves and treat imbalances due to stress and nervousness.

3. Is there a lot number and/or an expiration date on the product you are considering? This information provides important indicators of freshness. You also need to reference the lot number if you are requesting a certificate of analysis from the manufacturer or distributor.

4. Are you familiar with the manufacturer/brand? Dealing with reputable firms with a solid reputation is very important. Find out how long the company has been in business and if you can contact it with questions or concerns.

5. Is the label comprehensive? Be sure key components are not missing. For example, ingredients without amounts (for example, milligrams, micrograms, International Units) should be considered suspect.

Of course, it's also essential to understand what you're reading on the product label. For example, do you know the difference between concentration and potency? Following are brief definitions:

- **Concentration** refers to the amount of herb used compared to the amount of solvent. Obviously, a 1:1 concentration will be more powerful than a 1:10 concentration, which has more solvent than herbal material—10 times more solvent, to be exact.

- **Potency** can be more appropriately applied to the level of active constituents within a particular herb. Many experts believe that because standardized extracts have consistent potency, they provide a more consistent, accurate dosage and therapeutic effect.

RECOMMENDED DOSES. The recommended dose is 30 drops of the tincture or 250 to 500 mg of the capsule taken two to three times daily, or before bedtime for insomnia.

POTENTIAL SIDE EFFECTS. No known side effects are associated with taking Hops internally. There are rare cases of an allergic skin rash after handling Hops.

Rehmannia (Rehmannia glutinosa)

This perennial herb has light reddish-purple tubular flowers and a thick orange-yellow root.

APPLICATIONS. Rehmannia is used in Chinese herbal medicine for conditions such as irregular menses, palpitations, insomnia, dizziness, night sweats, vaginal dryness, and hot flashes.

HOW IT WORKS. I have not found any information on how Rehmannia works in Western medical literature although it likely benefits the adrenal glands. Its several uses, however, have been well-defined in terms of Chinese herbal therapy, and is said to have a "cooling" effect.

RECOMMENDED DOSES. This is another herb I would recommend only as part of a menopause formula. Doses of 100 to 200 mg per capsule are appropriate. It is best used under the care of a Chinese medicine practitioner or naturopathic physician.

POTENTIAL SIDE EFFECTS. Too high of a dosage can be hard on the digestive system as it can cause loose stools or a distended abdomen.

Red Clover (Trifolium pratense)

Red Clover, a popular grazing food for animals, may also provide health benefits to humans. The flower heads of this perennial herb are medicinal, whether dried or fresh. Although many different species exist, *trifolium pratense* is the one generally used for medicinal purposes. The name *trifolium* refers to the "three leaves" of the plant, which is a member of the pea family.

Historically, Red Clover is associated with cancer treatment. Today, it is emerging as an excellent source of isoflavones, estrogen-like substances that can play an important role during and after menopause. Studies indicate that Red Clover may also help prevent and treat heart disease and cancer.

APPLICATIONS

    Menopause. Red Clover is emerging as an alternative treatment for menopause. The phytoestrogens found in Red Clover can mimic some of the effects of estrogen, alleviating symptoms such as vaginal dryness and anxiety. Studies have shown mixed results concerning the ability of Red Clover extract to effectively reduce hot flashes and night sweats. Although Red Clover is clearly worth consideration, I don't consider it nearly as effective as Black Cohosh as a general treatment for menopausal symptoms.

- *Heart disease.* A study by Nestel et al. examined the effects of an isoflavone extract from Red Clover on the elasticity of the large arteries, which typically declines after menopause. Researchers found that the extract significantly improved arterial elasticity. The study concluded, ". . . [T]he findings indicate a potential new therapeutic approach for improved cardiovascular function after menopause." Red Clover extract has also been shown to increase beneficial HDL cholesterol.

- *Cancer.* Red Clover appears to block the growth of cancer in test-tube studies and has been historically used in herbal "anticancer" formulas.

HOW IT WORKS. Red Clover provides ten times as many estrogen isoflavones (daidzein and genistein) as soy. It also contains biochanin and formononetin, estrogenic isoflavones not found in soy.

RECOMMENDED DOSES. A typical dose of Red Clover comprises a tablet standardized to contain 40 mg of isoflavones (daidzein, genistein, biochanin, and formononetin) once or twice daily.

POTENTIAL SIDE EFFECTS. Red Clover is generally considered safe. However, pregnant or nursing women should not use Red Clover. Furthermore, women with a personal or family history of hormone-dependent cancers, such as breast cancer, should consult their physician before using Red Clover (although historically it has actually been used to treat these conditions). Individuals taking hormones or anticoagulants should also consult a physician before using Red Clover.

Burdock (Arctium lappa)

Burdock grows in hedges and ditches in Europe, parts of Asia, and North America. It is cultivated in Japan.

APPLICATIONS. Burdock is a traditional liver remedy. It is also used to treat digestive ailments, acne, psoriasis, respiratory troubles, *Candida,* and chronic fatigue syndrome.

HOW IT WORKS. By gently stimulating the liver, Burdock may reduce the irritability associated with hormonal imbalances. Burdock is also a natural diuretic (helps the body eliminate water), so it's helpful in decreasing bloating and breast tenderness. It appears to help clear the body of wastes.

RECOMMENDED DOSES. Adults should take 20 to 30 drops (0.5 ml) or 300 mg to 500 mg of the capsule form two to three times daily with meals.

POTENTIAL SIDE EFFECTS. Burdock is considered a safe herb. Rarely, direct contact with the skin may trigger a reaction.

THE ADVANTAGE OF FORMULAS

As you can see, there are many different herbs that can be used to help ease the symptoms of menopause. It would be neither practical nor cost-effective to purchase all the herbs mentioned in this chapter.

If you wanted to choose only one herb, I would recommend Black Cohosh because it has been the best studied and I have personally seen it help many women. In general, however, I recommend formulas that contain herbal blends. There are several good ones available.

OTHER HERBS

The herbs mentioned above are well-known for their ability to ease the transition into menopause. Here are other promising herbs you can use for specific symptoms:

- St. John's Wort *(Hypericum perforatum)* relieves mild, moderate, and possibly severe depression. Menopausal women may be more susceptible to mood disorders. In a 12-week study of 111 menopausal women, by Grube et al., nearly 80 percent reported improved psychological symptoms after treatment with St. John's Wort extract. In addition, patients reported improved sexual well-being.

People with serious depression may also benefit from using this herb. In a clinical trial by Vorbach et al., 209 patients with severe depression were given either St. John's Wort or the antidepressant drug imipramine. The researchers concluded that, at a dosage of 1,800 mg/day, St. John's Wort can be an effective treatment for severe depression.

It is generally advisable not to use St. John's Wort in combination with pharmaceutical antidepressants.

Dosage: For the treatment of depression, I recommend 300 mg of an extract to be taken three times daily. I recommend a standardized product containing 3% to 5% hyperforin and 0.3% hypericin. People usually notice improvement within two to six weeks. The tincture can also be used and is dosed at 30 drops (approximately 0.5 ml) three times daily.

▹ **Kava Root** *(Piper methysticum)* is an herbal nerve relaxer. In a double-blind, placebo-controlled study by Warnecke, 20 women with menopausal symptoms were given 100 mg of kavalactones (the active ingredients) daily. The women experienced benefits within the first week of treatment. Most of them reported improved mood and well-being, and less anxiety.

Kava may be recommended for adjustment disorder with anxiety, generalized anxiety disorder, obsessive–compulsive disorder, panic disorder, agoraphobia, social phobia, specific phobia, and post-traumatic stress disorder.

It is recommended that Kava Root not be used in combination with anti-anxiety pharmaceutical medications, or alcohol, or anyone with liver disease. It is best used on a short-term basis.

Dosage: A 250-mg capsule containing 30% kavalactones (equivalent to 75 mg kavalactones) can be taken two to three times daily.

➤ **Ginger** *(Zingiber officinale)* relieves indigestion, a common complaint among menopausal women. It works by promoting the release of saliva and gastric juices. Furthermore, Ginger stimulates digestion by increasing bile secretion. Increased bile secretion also helps relieve constipation and expel small gallstones. Ginger also helps substances move through the digestive tract, reducing irritation to the intestinal walls.

Dosage: Try a fresh cup of tea, or a 300- to 500-mg capsule, or 20 to 30 drops of tincture with meals.

➤ **Passionflower** *(Passiflora incarnata)* and **Valerian** *(Valeriana officinalis)* are both effective sleep aids. Menopausal women are especially susceptible to insomnia. In the United Kingdom, about 40 over-the-counter sedative formulas contain passionflower. Valerian is an approved, over-the-counter medicine for insomnia in Germany, Belgium, France, Switzerland, and Italy.

Dosages:

Passionflower: 300 to 500 mg of the capsule form, or 20 to 30 drops (0.5 ml) of the tincture form, or one cup of the tea, taken two to three times daily to calm the nervous system.

Valerian: 300 to 500 mg of the tincture capsule form, or 30 drops (0.5 ml) to 60 (1.0 ml) drops of the tincture, or one cup of the tea, taken two to three times daily.

NOTE: Valerian combines well with Scutellaria, Kava, Lemon Balm, and Passionflower for relaxation.

➤ **Siberian Ginseng** *(Eleutherococcus senticosus),* **Panax** *(Panax ginseng),* and **American Ginseng** *(P. quinquefolius)* promote energy and combat fatigue. Although all these forms of Ginseng have distinct characteristics, they also have many overlapping benefits. For example, they all affect the hypothalamus and pituitary, which in turn regulate adrenal function. Many individuals who suffer from fatigue have run-down adrenal glands.

NOT GOING COLD TURKEY

As you read about the potential of natural medicine, you may be tempted to switch from pharmaceutical remedies to plant medicines. If this is what you decide to do, be sure to consult a qualified healthcare practitioner first. Although herbal remedies provide gentle and effective healing to millions of women around the world, pharmaceuticals may be more appropriate in certain cases.

Some people are able to wean themselves from a pharmaceutical while starting an herbal medicine at small doses. This should only be done under a physician's supervision.

For example, I have had menopausal women wean from synthetic hormone replacement and replace them with herbal therapies or the sole use of natural progesterone.

There are many ways to do these switch-overs. For example, you can cut down the dose of the pharmaceutical by one-fourth every one to two weeks while simultaneously starting on an herb or desired natural product, building up the dosage over time as the pharmaceutical dosage is being lowered. Another technique is to start the natural product at full dosage while taking the pharmaceutical every other day, then reducing the pharmaceutical to every third day, and so on.

Although this approach works for many people, caution is necessary. First, withdrawing abruptly from a pharmaceutical agent can lead to withdrawal symptoms. I have talked to women who have been on synthetic hormone replacement for years who decide to suddenly stop cold turkey, and they felt like they were going crazy, as it is too much of a shock on the body.

Another factor to consider is potential interaction between pharmaceuticals and herbal extracts. For example, selective serotonin re-uptake inhibitors (SSRIs), such as Prozac® and Paxil®, may potentially interact with St. John's Wort. Both SSRIs and St. John's Wort appear to increase levels of serotonin in the brain. Serotonin is a key neurotransmitter that affects mood and appetite.

If you get too much serotonin in the brain, you may develop a condition known as Serotonin Syndrome. Symptoms include anxiety, rapid heartbeat, tremors, nervousness, euphoria, and confusion.

If you want to use pharmaceuticals and natural remedies in combination, do so only under the supervision of a qualified healthcare provider.

Panax Ginseng also appears to promote mental sharpness, which is helpful to women who complain of forgetfulness and absent-mindedness during menopause. A double-blind, cross-over study on university students in Italy, by D'Angelo et al., compared Panax Ginseng to a placebo. Ginseng was found to enhance attention, improve mental arithmetic and logical deduction, integrate brain–body function, and decrease reaction time to sounds. The Ginseng group also reported a greater sense of well-being. However, American Ginseng is the preferred type of Ginseng, as it has a "cooling effect." Siberian Ginseng can also be used as it supports adrenal function and has a "neutral" effect on temperature regulation. Panax Ginseng, on the other hand, is best used under the guidance of a Chinese herbal practitioner or naturopathic doctor as it is a very warming herb, and in some cases may worsen hot flashes and other symptoms of menopause.

Dosages:

Panax Ginseng (best used under care of experienced herbal practitioner): Standardized between 4% to 7% ginsenosides. The dose is 100 mg two to three times daily.

Siberian Ginseng: Standardized capsule extract containing 0.4% eleutherosides at 300 mg two to three times daily.

American Ginseng: 1,000 to 2,000 mg daily of the capsule or 30 drops (1 ml) to 60 drops (2 ml) of the tincture taken two to three times daily.

ᴥ **Bilberry** *(Vaccinium myrtillus)* and **Horse Chestnut** *(Aesculus hippocastanum)* help ward off varicose veins. Hormonal imbalances are believed to contribute to this condition. Bilberry stimulates the development of new capillaries, strengthens capillary walls, and improves overall circulatory health. Aescin, the active compound in Horse Chestnut, bolsters capillary cells and reduces fluid leakage.

In North America, more than one-half of all adults over 50—mostly women—are afflicted with varicose veins. Risk factors for getting them include obesity, a family history of varicose veins, pregnancy, hormonal changes, and jobs that require a lot of standing or lifting.

Dosages:

Bilberry: 160 mg twice daily containing 25% anthocyanosides extract.

Horse Chestnut: 300 mg twice daily (equivalent to 100 mg of the active constituent aescin daily).

ᴥ **Cranberry** *(Vaccinium macrocarpon)* protects against urinary tract infections, a common malady among menopausal women. Cranberry juice helps prevent bacteria from sticking to the walls and lining of the bladder and urinary tract. A 1998 study in *The New England Journal of Medicine* demonstrated that cranberry prevents the fimbriae (analogous to arms and hands of bacteria) from attaching to the urinary tract walls. It prevents urinary tract infections more effectively than either orange juice or grapefruit juice. It is also available in standardized tablet or capsule form.

Cranberries may also protect against heart disease. A study by Wilson et al. examined the effects of cranberry extract on low-density lipoprotein (LDL) oxidation. Researchers concluded that "cranberry extracts have the ability to inhibit the oxidative modification of LDL particles."

Dosage: I recommend 8 ounces of the unsweetened juice two to four times daily for women with a history of urinary tract infections. Follow directions on label for the capsule or tablet form, as products vary in their potency.

ᴥ **Milk Thistle** *(Silybum marianum)* and **Dandelion Root** *(Taraxacum officinale)* both support the liver, which metabolizes hormones. Milk Thistle has been shown to prevent liver damage and help restore liver function. Dandelion also helps improve the liver's ability to detoxify.

In our modern world, the liver is under constant assault from environmental toxins, alcohol, and other drugs.

Dosages for women requiring liver support:

Milk Thistle: A 200- to 250-mg capsule of a standardized extract (80% to 85% silymarin) three times daily.

Dandelion Root: A 200- to 250-mg capsule or 20 to 30 drops of tincture capsule with each meal.

❧ **Tribulus** *(Tribulus terrestris),* also known as Puncture Vine, and Damiana (Turnera diffusa), have both been historically used by herbalists for low libido, although scientific research is lacking. Dosage is 500 mg three times daily.

4

$\mathcal{C}$USTOMIZING YOUR
HORMONE REPLACEMENT

$\mathcal{L}$et's reiterate an important fact that is often mysteriously absent from pharmaceutical hormone propaganda: *Your body produces hormones (estrogen, progesterone, and so on) in glands / organs other than the ovaries.* If it didn't, and the ovaries quit producing hormones altogether (ovary hormone production actually slows down, rather than shutting down completely), menopausal women would become "vegetables." After all, without hormones, a body can't function. So in the infinite wisdom of our Creator, a backup or secondary system was created to help us out. I have already mentioned how the adrenal glands produce precursor molecules for DHEA and so forth. The brain, skin, body fat, and nerves can and do produce hormones as well.

This has important implications for hormone replacement. Since we're not trying to replenish a completely dormant system, we should use only the specific hormones needed, at the lowest dose necessary, and for the shortest possible time. Otherwise, we might run into problems with toxicity and undesired side effects. So we need to customize hormone replacement to specifically meet the needs of individuals.

If you're menotype C, for example, then you will definitely have a requirement for hormones. Depending on your situation as a menotype B, you may also require the use of certain hormones such as natural progesterone, DHEA, or others. If you're menotype A, you also should pay close attention to this chapter, especially the information on thyroid dysfunction, which affects so many women over age 30.

ASSESSING YOUR HORMONE LEVELS

There are three keys to diagnosing perimenopause and menopause: age, symptoms, and hormone levels. Of these, measuring hormone levels gives the most accurate assessment. Unfortunately, the most common way of measuring them—blood tests—doesn't necessarily give the best answers.

For example, elevated blood values of the pituitary hormones FSH and LH suggest that a woman is menopausal. However, the levels can fluctuate widely during perimenopause. Thus, one cannot say for sure that a woman is perimenopausal with a single measurement of FSH and LH.

Beyond FSH and LH, doctors often order standard blood hormone tests for total amounts of estrogen, progesterone, and sometimes testosterone. While this gives a "ballpark" assessment, it's not terribly accurate. Why? Because these tests usually measure the bound (inactive) form of the hormone. You can have massive amounts of hormones floating around your bloodstream bound to protein molecules (globulin), but unless they become unbound, they cannot enter tissues and cells. They're like a pile of quarters you've left in your top drawer at home. You can't spend or do much else with them while they remain in that drawer. When you need to use a public telephone, the quarters in your purse are the ones that count.

Since the bound hormones in your body don't do anything, it makes far more sense to measure unbound, free hormones—also referred to as biologically active hormones. To do this, your doctor will need to order specific tests for "free" levels.

Unfortunately for perimenopausal women, even these tests don't really give us the answers we need, because results will vary with the time of day, or even the time of month the test is done. How, then, are we to get the measurements we're looking for? Many holistic doctors prefer another system of hormone testing that uses saliva samples instead of blood.

THYROID POWER

The bowtie-shaped thyroid gland is located in front of the neck below the voice box. This gland produces and secrets two hormones known as T3 (triiodothyronine) and T4 (thyroxine). Your thyroid gland makes these hormones from iodine you ingest in your foods. Thyroid hormones have many powerful effects on your body. First, it controls the metabolism of your cells so that they produce energy. This is important because a low-functioning thyroid can lead to fatigue and weight gain. Thyroid hormones also have effects on carbohydrate metabolism, fat metabolism, and vitamin metabolism. Irregular menstrual bleeding or no cycle at all can be due to low thyroid. Among men, low thyroid can lead to complete loss of libido and high thyroid can lead to impotence. High cholesterol and triglycerides can also be a sign of low thyroid function, as thyroid hormone influences the liver metabolism of these substances. There is a direct connection between the heart and thyroid function. Thyroid hormones influence heart rate and the strength of the heartbeat.

Classic symptoms of low thyroid function include one or more of the following: fatigue, dry skin, constipation, and poor memory. It can also cause your skin, hair, and nails to become rough, dry, brittle, and slow growing. In addition, depression can be caused by an underfunctioning thyroid gland. Infertility can be the result of low thyroid function in women of childbearing age. Joint pain and increased cholesterol levels can also be the result of low thyroid function.

There are various reasons for the thyroid becoming "sluggish." Environmental toxins are suspect, as are the effects of stress, and anxiety can lower stimulation of the thyroid by the pituitary gland. Estrogen dominance appears to inhibit thyroid function. We have found that by balancing estrogen and progesterone ratios, thyroid function often improves. Adrenal hormone balance also is helpful, especially when DHEA levels are normalized.

For thyroid hormone replacement, many holistic doctors prefer more balanced hormones, such as Armour Thyroid® or Thyrolar® to common medications such as Synthroid®.

THE NEXT GENERATION OF HORMONE TESTING: SALIVA TESTING

Saliva testing is accurate, dependable, and simple. A patient takes home a hormone profile kit, which contains plastic tubes for collecting saliva. At specified times over a period of a day or days (depending on which hormone profile is being used), a patient spits into a tube and marks the time and date. Sounds quite simple, and it is. There are several advantages to saliva hormone testing:

1. It measures "free" levels of a hormone.

2. Multiple samples can be easily obtained throughout the day or week. This allows for a more accurate assessment than a one-shot blood draw.

3. It's cost-effective.

4. Patients show good compliance, as the test can be done at home or work. As an added bonus, one does not get poked with a needle.

When a saliva sample is sent to a lab, the technicians add antibodies and radioactive markers to the saliva mixture. These adhere to the free hormones so that a value can be measured. This type of testing is known as Radio Immuno Assay (RIA).

Several studies have validated the effectiveness and accuracy of saliva hormone testing, and currently a huge number of doctors have begun using it. In five years, it's likely to be the method of choice throughout the healthcare community.

Saliva hormone testing kits are available from holistic doctors, pharmacies, health food stores, and on the Internet. Make sure to use reputable companies (see Resources) and work with a knowledgeable doctor to help you interpret the results if you do the testing on your own.

NOTE: Women on hormone-therapy will have altered saliva hormone results which must be taken into consideration when analyzing the results.

DON'T TAKE HORMONES YOU DON'T NEED

Just having low levels of hormones does not mean you absolutely need hormone replacement therapy (HRT). Hormone levels always drop during menopause. This is normal. But if you have no symptoms or major risk factors (for example, osteoporosis), there's really no reason for you to put extra hormones into your system. Only extreme deficiencies coupled with problematic symptoms or risk factors require HRT.

URINE TESTING

Urinalysis is yet another way to measure hormone levels. Some doctors and researchers feel it is more accurate than standard blood hormone tests, as it can measure free hormone levels. The downside of this type of testing, however, is the inconvenience of collecting urine over a 24-hour period. I prefer saliva to urinalysis testing for hormone levels, but it's really a matter of personal choice. See the Resources for labs that specialize in urine hormone testing.

BLOOD TESTS

Specialized blood tests that measure hormone levels can be helpful for menopausal or postmenopausal women. For example, we often use one blood test that measures the three estrogens (progesterone, testosterone, DHEA) and estrogen metabolites such as 16 alpha-hydroxyestrogen, a metabolite associated with increased breast cancer risk. Currently there are no saliva tests that measure the levels of 16 alpha-hydroxyestrogen.

BIOIDENTICAL HORMONES: THE LOGICAL CHOICE

Many years ago the term "bioidentical hormones" came into use with reference to hormones that are identical to those produced by the

TESTING IS ONLY ONE PIECE OF THE PUZZLE

Hormone testing allows a doctor to identify which hormones are at very low levels and to get an idea of what dosages to prescribe. However, lab tests should not be used as an absolute guide for dosage recommendations. How a patient feels while on hormone therapy is very important and should not be disregarded, even if lab values are "normal." Communication between physician and patient is important. If the patient says she's not feeling quite right, the doctor should take that into account when adjusting her dosage. He should also have a baseline measurement, taken during perimenopause, against which he can compare test results taken throughout the menopausal transition.

human body. (This term was "coined" and trademarked by Marcus Laux, N.D., who has given us permission to use this trademarked term throughout this book.) Bioidentical hormones are made from plant substances found in soybeans or Mexican wild yams. The three different estrogens and progesterone can all be duplicated in this way.

These plant-derived hormones are often called "natural" hormones, but that confuses some patients and some doctors as well. After all, plants are found in nature, but so are the horses that produce "synthetic" hormones. The important fact is that the estrogens in Premarin® and other synthetic patented brands are not identical to those found in your body.

Let's take a closer look at what these hormones are and what they do.

Estrogen

No other female hormone gets more mainstream attention than estrogen. Estrogen is important for menstruation and reproduction throughout a woman's life. It gives women their secondary sex characteristics and has effects on their mood, libido, bone density, cardiovascular health, and brain function.

Actually, the body produces three different types of estrogen: estrone, estradiol, and estriol, each with different functions.

- **Estrone** becomes the primary estrogen when ovarian production of estradiol decreases during menopause. It is synthesized in the ovaries and fat tissue.

- **Estradiol** is considered the most potent of the three estrogens. Levels typically decline during menopause as ovarian production decreases.

- **Estriol** is the least potent estrogen but is thought to exert a protective effect against estrogen-associated cancers. Some studies have shown it to be helpful for hot flashes and to increase bone density. It is not nearly so well studied as estradiol for these purposes. The placenta secretes the highest amounts of estriol during pregnancy.

HOW NATURAL ARE "NATURAL" HORMONES?

A clinic's manager once told me about a pharmaceutical sales representative who came to her clinic for an unscheduled visit to talk about Premarin®. She politely informed this representative that the doctors had no time to talk that day and that natural estrogen was their hormone of choice. The pharmaceutical representative was annoyed that no one would meet with her, and in a rude manner stated, "Well, Premarin® is natural." The clinic manager replied, "Yes, it is natural—for horses!" and escorted her out of the clinic.

You may wonder why a pharmaceutical company would manufacture anything but a bioidentical hormone. It's all about patents and business. For a pharmaceutical company to patent a hormone, it cannot be identical to a substance found in nature (or the body). The hormone must be chemically altered. As you may have guessed, this causes inherent flaws in the synthetic hormone right from the start. Our bodies were not designed to metabolize synthetic hormones and their metabolites efficiently. For these reasons, nonidentical hormones appear to be more toxic to cell DNA and liver than bioidentical ones.

Classic symptoms of estrogen deficiency include hot flashes, night sweats, and especially vaginal dryness and thinning of the vaginal walls. Recurring urinary tract infections or incontinence may also be connected to low estrogen. Mood swings and irritability may be signs as well. Other symptoms can also be present and vary depending on the individual.

This does not mean that estrogen needs to be used if you have these symptoms. If you are a menotype C, then natural progesterone by itself may work well for you (remembering that progesterone is a precursor molecule for estrogen). Only hormone testing will tell you if a major deficiency is present.

Classic symptoms of too much estrogen (generally due to hormone replacement) can include nausea and vomiting, breast tenderness or enlargement, fluid retention, increased growth of uterine fibroids, bloating, vaginal bleeding, recurring yeast infections, headaches, and spotty darkening of the skin, especially on the face.

NATURAL PRESCRIPTIONS OF ESTROGEN. More and more doctors are prescribing bioidentical estrogens. Initially many doctors prescribed what was known as "tri-estrogen." This was the formulation concept of Jonathan Wright, M.D., who felt it most closely mimicked a woman's hormonal physiology. It was a compounded formulation (meaning made up by a pharmacy) that comprised 80% estriol, 10% estradiol, and 10% estrone. The dosage equivalent to 0.625 mg of Premarin® is 1 mg estriol, 0.125 mg estradiol, and 0.125 mg estrone. This dosage is given twice daily. Holistic doctors often use tri-estrogen in combination with natural progesterone to maintain balance.

Another formulation, known as bi-estrogen, has also become popular, as it does not contain estrone. Research is showing that some of the metabolites of estrone (16 alpha-hydroxyestrone) may be associated with an increased risk of breast cancer. An equivalent dose to 0.625 mg of Premarin® is 2.5 mg given twice daily.

Last, some practitioners prescribe estriol by itself to relieve menopausal symptoms. The theory is that it may have the least potential

THE DARK SIDE OF PREMARIN®

Premarin® is the most widely prescribed hormone for women and one of the most prescribed drugs overall in the U.S., but its use horrifies many holistic doctors. Here's why.

According to the *Physician's Desk Reference,* Premarin® "contains estrone, **equilin,** and 17-**dihydroequilin,** together with smaller amounts of 17-estradiol, **equilenin,** and 17-**dihydroequilenin.**"

Please note that all the words in boldface are hormones that occur naturally only in horse urine (*equine* refers to horses and thus all the horse hormones in Premarin® are derived from this word). According to one published study, equilin and equilenin make up approximately 20 percent of Premarin®, quite a substantial amount.

It is known that estrogen stimulates cell growth and pharmaceutical use increases the risk of breast and endometrial cancer. Studies have shown that the metabolites of horse estrogens found in Premarin® damage cell DNA. Remember, one of the leading theories as to why cancer develops is that damaged cell DNA (the genetic code of cells that controls cell division) leads to cancer formation. Several *in vitro* studies have shown that Premarin® metabolites damage cell DNA and, according to researchers, may have carcinogenic effects. It appears that these toxic metabolites of Premarin® may be partly to blame for users' increased risk of endometrial and breast cancer.

for side effects. A few studies have shown it to be helpful for hot flashes and bone density, but much more research is needed. Holistic doctors generally prefer to apply estriol to the vagina to relieve dryness and thinning, as well as urinary frequency.

An average oral dosage of estriol is 2 mg per day, but dosage can range up to 8 mg daily. A typical dosage of vaginal cream (at a concentration of 0.5 mg per gram of cream) is to insert 1 gram of cream daily for one to two weeks and then to repeat the application once or twice every week after that.

MELATONIN—SNOOZING ... AND MUCH MORE

Melatonin is a hormone that promotes sound sleep. It is mainly produced by the pineal gland, a small pea-size structure located in the center of the brain. Darkness activates an increase in melatonin production, and light causes a reduction. It is a popular over-the-counter hormone used for people with insomnia, those adjusting to a "graveyard shift," and those adjusting to a new time zone to prevent "jet lag." It is also showing some promise as an adjunctive therapy for people receiving chemotherapy and radiation for hormone-dependent cancers, such as breast cancer and prostate cancer. Researchers are also investigating its role in protecting against radiation damage.

The production of melatonin does not necessarily decrease as one ages. Therefore, if one uses it, I recommend that the lowest possible dosage be taken. Many people get relief from insomnia at very low dosages (0.3 to 0.5 mg). I find it rare for patients to need more than 3 mg to promote sleep. Since it is a powerful hormone, I generally recommend it as a last resort. Try other therapies for insomnia first, such as the herbs Passionflower, Kava, or Valerian Root. There are many good homeopathic insomnia formulas as well.

Progesterone

This hormone is involved in regulating the menstrual cycle and reproductive function (maintains the endometrium when implantation has occurred). Progesterone is mainly secreted by the ovary during the second half of the menstrual cycle. The drop in progesterone near the end of the cycle is what starts menstruation. The adrenal glands synthesize it during and after menopause. High amounts are produced during pregnancy to maintain the endometrium and maintain the pregnancy.

Progesterone has several metabolic functions in the body before and after menopause, which include mood regulation, circulation, blood-sugar balance, water-balance regulation, bone growth, libido, and thyroid and adrenal function. Several hormones, such as estrogen, testosterone, androstenedione, cortisol, and aldosterone, are formed from progesterone. One of its main functions is to maintain balance with estrogen so as to prevent estrogen dominance and thus side effects such as PMS, breast cancer, and so on.

DEFINING PROGESTERONE

Different books and resource materials use various terms when it comes to progesterone. The following brief glossary will help clarify any misunderstanding:

Progestogen—A substance that possesses progestational activity. This can be either synthetic or bioidentical progesterone.

Progestin—Synthetic version of progesterone, altered so that it is not identical to progesterone found in the human body.

Progesterone—A natural hormone found in the body or a bioidentical hormone made from plants.

Classic symptoms of progesterone deficiency include PMS, premenstrual migraine headaches, irregular and heavy menstrual cycles, anxiety, insomnia, hot flashes, cyclical depression, and painful or fibrocystic breasts. Other indicators of progesterone deficiency may include ovarian cysts, infertility, yeast infections, menopausal weight gain, hair loss, low libido, endometriosis, and osteoporosis.

Symptoms of too much progesterone can include breast swelling and tenderness, drowsiness, headaches, and mood changes such as depression and irritability.

Progesterone is a hormone to consider for menotype B's and is essential for menotype C's. The question is whether to use synthetic or the bioidentical (natural) form, and which route of administration to use (for example, transdermal, oral, etc.).

WHAT'S THE DEAL WITH PROVERA®? Provera®, as well as the trade names Amen® and Cycrin®, are progestins. As I described earlier, this is another way to say synthetic progesterone. Similar to synthetic estrogen, the progesterone molecule has been altered so that it can be patented, but in doing so it becomes a chemical that's foreign to the body. Synthetic progesterone is technically known as medroxyprogesterone acetate, which is also the form of progesterone found in the commonly prescribed hormone replacement products known as Prempro® and Premphase.®

Side effects associated with synthetic progesterone products such as Provera® include blood clots, fluid retention, breast tenderness, acne, hair loss, hirsuitism, breakthrough bleeding (when a woman doesn't have a cycle and then starts uterine bleeding), nausea, jaundice, depression, edema, weight change, and anaphylaxis. Studies on beagle dogs with medroxyprogesterone acetate showed that some developed breast nodules, some of which were cancerous.

SYNTHETIC PROGESTERONE AND BREAST CANCER. The primary purpose of using synthetic progesterone is to prevent uterine cancer among women on estrogen replacement. However, a study of postmenopausal women who were current or recent users of the combination of synthetic estrogen and synthetic progesterone had a relatively higher risk of breast cancer than women who took only estrogen. In fact, postmenopausal women who used this combination of synthetic estrogen and progesterone in the past four years had a 40-percent higher risk as compared to women who never used hormone replacement therapy.

GROWTH HORMONE

Growth hormone does just what its name implies: It promotes growth of the body tissues, including bone and lean muscle tissue. It has become popular among anti-aging enthusiasts and athletes. This hormone is produced by the pituitary gland and then metabolized by the liver to create IGF-1 (insulin growthlike factor-1) and other growth factors. Although it holds promise for such conditions as fatigue, osteoporosis, and heart disease, many doctors feel more long-term studies need to be done before it is routinely used. Exercise is one way to naturally stimulate the endogenous production of growth hormone. Side effects of too much growth hormone may include diabetes, carpal tunnel syndrome, arthritis, and cancer. This hormone must be used under the guidance of a knowledgeable doctor.

The Nurses' Health Study, which involved close to 122,000 women, found that women who took only estrogen had a 36-percent increase in breast cancer risk, those on the combination of estrogen and progestin had a 50-percent increased risk, and those on progestin alone had a 240-percent increase. Again, this was a study with only synthetic hormones. Not all studies have, of course, been this negative, but remember, the results of this 1995 study involved a large number of women.

Unfortunately, no studies have been done on the use of natural estrogen and natural progesterone with regard to any associated risk of breast cancer. My experience and those of my colleagues is that these natural versions are much safer. Follow-up testing of our own patients shows that hormones come into a more natural balance with the use of bioidentical versions.

SYNTHETIC PROGESTERONE AND CARDIOVASCULAR HEALTH. Progesterone is available in many different forms. Obviously I recommend bioidentical progesterone. Natural progesterone creams are available over the counter without a prescription. Virtually every health food store carries them and more pharmacies are making them available to their female customers.

THE OLD IN A NEW WAY

Pharmaceutical companies now make the use of hormone combinations more convenient. Combination packages that contain estrogen and progesterone are becoming popular prescriptions for physicians. Prempro®, Premphase®, Ortho-Prefest®, and FemHRT® are all combination drugs. Unfortunately, none of these combinations contain both bioidentical estrogen and progesterone.

Natural progesterone cream works very well for the relief of perimenopausal and menopausal symptoms. Dr. John Lee, a retired gynecologist, has shared his successful experience with natural progesterone through his books and seminars. He feels the transdermal natural progesterone is the best route of administration and cites many case examples of success that range from reducing PMS and alleviating menopausal symptoms, to increasing bone density.

More research is needed to clarify the best application of natural progesterone. Yet many holistic doctors and practitioners find excellent results with therapeutic natural progesterone creams. A study completed by St. Luke's Hospital in Bethlehem, PA, found that using progesterone cream prevented build up of the endometrium (uterine lining) among postmenopausal women who were taking synthetic estrogen (Premarin®). This is good news as it was previously unknown whether these creams had this benefit.

Various brands of creams differ in their potency. Look for products that contain 960 mg per two ounces. Thus, one-quarter teaspoon of natural progesterone cream is equivalent to 20 mg of progesterone.

For good absorption, natural progesterone cream is best applied to areas of skin with high capillary density. These include the chest, inner arms, neck, face, and palms if they are not callused.

- **Perimenopausal:** Women who are still having a menses should discontinue use during the five to seven days of the menses.

- **Menopausal:** Apply one-quarter teaspoon (20 mg) of natural progesterone twice daily for two to three weeks a month.

- **Postmenopausal:** Apply one-quarter teaspoon one to two times daily for three continuous weeks each month.

NOTE: For women who desire to remain on Premarin® and wish to use natural progesterone, apply one-quarter teaspoon twice daily on the days the Premarin® is taken. The dosage of Premarin® often needs to be reduced (sometimes by 50% or more) when it is used with natural progesterone, so consult with your doctor about dosage issues.

The dosages given here are general guidelines that work well for most women. However, as I have emphasized in this book, all women are biochemically unique and you need to find the right dosage for you. This is best done by working with a holistic doctor, finding the dose that works best for you. Salivary or other types of hormone testing will help guide you as well.

COMPOUNDING PHARMACIES

In the United States and Canada, specialized pharmacies known as "compounding pharmacies" offer bioidentical hormones through a doctor's prescription. Their pharmacists are specially trained in formulating natural hormones, and they can fill hormone prescriptions formulated to suit the unique needs of each patient. Most cities have compounding pharmacies. If your doctor is not familiar with bioidentical hormones and would like more information about the nearest compounding pharmacy, have him or her contact one of the referral agencies in the Resources section. Also, the contacts in the Resources can help you find a doctor knowledgeable in natural hormone replacement.

SHE TRIED IT

Jenny, a 50-year-old, started using natural progesterone cream on her own to relieve hot flashes, night sweats, insomnia, and other related menopausal symptoms. She told us she had been using the cream for almost two months and was not noticing any reduction in her menopausal symptoms. I examined the cream she was using and found that it contained only about 4 mg per quarter teaspoon. No wonder she wasn't experiencing any improvement. We then recommended Jenny use a cream that contained 20 mg per quarter teaspoon and she found her menopausal symptoms started to subside over the next four weeks.

There are several prescription forms of natural progesterone that work quite well. With regard to the capsule form, many doctors use what is known as oral micronized progesterone (OMP). This makes the progesterone much more absorbable. One of the benefits of OMP is that it has been shown to prevent build up of the endometrium in women who are using estrogen. Nor does it have the negative effects on lipids that synthetic progesterone has been shown to have.

The typical dose of OMP for a perimenopausal woman on continuous estrogen therapy who is still having a cycle is 100 mg twice daily or 200 mg once daily 12 days per month. Another option for a woman on estrogen therapy is to take 50 mg of OMP twice daily or 100 mg once daily for three weeks on and one week off (stop during menses). For postmenopausal women on continuous estrogen, the dosage is 50 mg of OMP twice daily or 100 mg once daily taken on a continuous basis.

There are several other forms of application of natural progesterone that include capsules, drops, vaginal gel, transdermal gel, and many other forms. Your doctor can work with a compounding pharmacy to find the best dosage regimen for you.

BIRTH CONTROL FOR SYMPTOM CONTROL?

Birth-control pills are sometimes recommended during perimenopause to help control heavy menstrual flow and irregular cycles. Although an option, it makes more sense to use herbal, homeopathic, or even natural progesterone to smooth out irregular cycles. Birth-control pills are composed of different formulations of synthetic estrogen and synthetic progesterone.

Testosterone

Although thought of as a male hormone, testosterone is an important hormone for women as well. Some women experience a rapid decline of their testosterone levels during menopause, while for others it remains in the normal range or increases slightly. Again, hormone testing is the only way to know. Some of the key functions of testosterone include libido, bone density, skin health, and cardiovascular health. In combination with estrogen, testosterone has been shown to help decrease hot flashes as well as increase sex drive. Also, in combination with estrogen, studies show that it can increase bone density more effectively than estrogen alone. I will have more to say about this in Chapter 11.

Symptoms of testosterone deficiency may include a low libido, vaginal wall thinning, and decreased energy. Women taking too much testosterone may experience acne, mood changes, deepening of voice, and increased facial hair.

As with other hormones, testosterone is available by prescription in the synthetic form (methyltestosterone) and the bioidentical form (testosterone). Testosterone cream applied to the genital area has become popular for improving sexual response as well as a treatment for vaginal wall thinning and improving lubrication. This is done through a prescription with a 0.5%, 1%, or 2% cream applied to the vulva twice weekly or as directed by your physician.

BOOSTING TESTOSTERONE

One way to increase testosterone levels is through the supplemental use of DHEA, which acts as a precursor to testosterone. Often 20 to 50 mg of DHEA is sufficient to elevate testosterone levels. This is a more "gentle" way to increase levels and improve a sagging libido. For some women it works well, while others derive more benefit from actual testosterone. This should all be done under the guidance of a knowledgeable physician.

For internal use, holistic doctors often have testosterone made by a compounding pharmacy and mixed (0.5 to 1.0 mg) with estrogen and progesterone as a cream or gel. It is also available in capsule or sublingual form.

CHART OF HORMONES

ESTROGENS

Product name	Bioidentical	Comments
Premarin®	no	
Cenestin®	no	similar composition to Premarin®
Estrace®	yes	contains estradiol
Gynodiol®	yes	contains estradiol
Ortho-Est®	no	

Product name	Bioidentical	Comments
Ogen®	no	
Menest®	no	
Estratab®	no	
Estraderm®	yes	patch containing estradiol
Vivelle®	yes	patch containing estradiol
Vivelle Dot®	yes	patch containing estradiol
Climara®	yes	patch containing estradiol
Akora®	yes	patch containing estradiol
E2 111®	yes	patch containing estradiol
Esclim®	yes	patch containing estradiol
Estring®	yes	vaginal silicone ring containing estradiol
Ortho Dienestrol®	no	vaginal estrogen cream
Vagifem®	no	vaginal tablet
Tri-estrogen®	yes	contains estrone, estradiol, estriol made by compounding pharmacy
Biestrogen®	yes	contains estriol and estradiol made by compounding pharmacy
Estradiol®	yes	made by compounding pharmacy
Estriol®	yes	made by compounding pharmacy

PROGESTINS/PROGESTERONE

Product name	Bioidentical	Comments
Provera®	no	
Cycrin®	no	
Amen®	no	
Prometrium®	yes	do not use if allergic to peanut
Aygestin®	no	
Nor-QD® (norethindrone)	no	birth control pill sometimes used for HRT
Micronor®	no	
Megace®	no	not generally used for HRT but as a palliative treatment for breast or endometrial cancer
Crinone®	yes	vaginal gel

Product name	Bioidentical	Comments
Natural Micronized Progesterone	yes	
Progesterone cream	yes	made by many different companies or compounding pharmacy

COMBINATION ESTROGEN/PROGESTIN OR PROGESTERONE

Product name	Bioidentical	Comments
Prempro®	no	contains Premarin® and synthetic progesterone
FemHRT®	no	
Ortho-Prefest®	yes/no	bioidentical estrogen (estradiol) with synthetic progesterone
Activella®	yes/no	bioidentical estrogen (estradiol) with synthetic progesterone
Premphase®	no	contains Premarin® and synthetic progesterone
Combi Patch®	yes/no	bioidentical estrogen with synthetic progesterone
Triestrogen with progesterone	yes	
Biestrogen with progesterone	yes	
Estradiol with progesterone	yes	
Estriol with progesterone	yes	

TESTOSTERONE PREPARATIONS

Product name	Bioidentical	Comments
Estratest®, Estratest HS®	no	synthetic estrogen and synthetic testosterone
Menogen®, Menogen HS®	no	synthetic estrogen and synthetic testosterone
Testosterone	yes	made by compounding pharmacy
Methyltestosterone	no	

DHEA

Dehydroepiandrosterone is the most abundant of the sex steroids produced by the adrenal glands and to a lesser extent by the ovaries. It is a precursor to other sex hormones such as testosterone and estrogen.

DHEA has many direct effects on the body. As with cortisol, it works to decrease the body's resistance to stress and disease. It appears to have a protective effect on the bones and cardiovascular system (lowers LDL cholesterol). DHEA acts as a balancer to cortisol (high levels of cortisol lead to immune system breakdown). Menopausal symptoms result from deficient DHEA levels since it is a precursor to estrogen and testosterone. It is important for brain function and is found in high concentration in the brain.

We commonly find low levels in menopausal women who have been under chronic bouts of stress in recent years. Saliva testing will dictate what dosage should be used, but in women who are deficient, we usually start at 10 mg to 25 mg and adjust the dosage as dictated by follow up testing. When used in physiological doses, DHEA appears to be very safe. One of the first symptoms of too much DHEA supplementation is back or facial acne, which goes away when the dosage is reduced.

Cortisol

Cortisol has long been recognized as a "stress hormone," because it helps to negate the effects of physical and mental stress. It is also produced by the adrenal glands and has several functions that include carbohydrate, protein, and fat metabolism. It is intricately involved in blood-sugar metabolism and works to reduce inflammatory states in the body.

Long-term elevation of cortisol is associated with several imbalances and disease processes, including chronic fatigue, impaired blood-sugar levels, depression, memory impairment, insomnia, decreased immune function, obesity, high blood pressure, heart disease, hypothyroidism, menstrual disorders, irregular menstrual cycles, and osteoporosis. Also, decreased levels may result from prolonged stimulation and "burnout" from stress.

HOW TO TAKE HORMONES

There are many different ways to administer hormones. Which is the best one? There's no single answer. I have seen some patients do well on creams and others do better with sublingual or other forms. By working with a knowledgeable doctor and compounding pharmacy, you can get the prescription that works best for you. Here are the various ways you might try:

- Oral—tablets or capsules
- Transdermal—creams, gels, patches
- Sublingual—drops, pellets
- Injection
- Intravaginal—creams or rings
- Pellet implants
- Suppositories
- Lozenges

Deficient levels also predispose a person to many of the same illnesses as listed for long-term cortisol elevation. As with other hormones, a balanced range is required for good health.

You can lower elevated levels through exercise and a hormone-balancing program, which may include DHEA, herbs such as Ginseng, and various stress-reduction techniques.

Deficient levels may be helped with the use of Ginseng (especially Chinese and Siberian Ginseng), Licorice Root, glandulars, vitamin C, zinc, pantothenic acid, vitamin B12, and, in more severe cases, small amounts (physiological amounts) of cortisol as prescribed by a physician.

Diet and lifestyle play important roles in the health of the adrenal glands. A diet high in refined sugars, animal protein, or stimulating substances such as caffeine and nicotine wreak havoc on the adrenals. Too little sleep, no exercise, dysfunctional work/social relationships, and lack of spiritual focus can all stress the adrenals as well.

Pregnenelone

Pregnenelone is a precursor of the steroid hormones. It appears to have benefit for depression, memory, and rheumatoid arthritis. Many practitioners find that using pregnenelone alone in menopausal women is not very therapeutic, but when combined with other hormones, it provides a noticeable benefit. Although it is available over the counter, I do not recommend its use without the guidance of a knowledgeable doctor. A typical starting dosage would be 50 mg to 100 mg.

Androstenedione

Women in postmenopause secrete approximately five times more androstenedione than do women in perimenopause. Androstenedione serves as a major precursor hormone as ovarian production decreases, so some doctors may include it in a comprehensive hormone replacement program. Although it's a popular supplement among male bodybuilders (theoretically as a testosterone precursor), studies have actually shown it increases estrogen rather than testosterone levels.

5

$\mathcal{N}$UTRITION

$\mathcal{Y}$ou are what you eat. It's an old saw, but it contains a lot of truth, especially for women who are going through menopause.

Good nutrition is the very foundation of the menotype-A program, and when consistently followed, it reduces the chances that you'll need medications or supplements for menopause-related health problems in the future. Women who are menotype B will notice a reduction of symptoms once they begin avoiding "unfriendly foods" and incorporate "friendly foods" into their diet on a regular basis. Women who are menotype C should pay particular attention to the foods that affect bone health because of their osteoporosis risk.

GUIDELINES TO A MENOPAUSE-FRIENDLY FOOD DIET

Vegetables, fruits, nuts, seeds, and whole grains are all sources of the naturally occurring hormone balancers known as phytosterols. These plant chemicals are structurally similar to human hormones and appear to fit neatly into human hormone receptor sites. Researchers are currently investigating the balancing effects of phytosterols on estrogen and progesterone levels in the body.

Plant foods are also potent sources of phytonutrients that play an important role as antioxidants, immune enhancement, detoxification, and ultimately as hormone balancers.

Unfortunately, the average American woman doesn't enjoy the advantages of phytosterols and phytonutrients because she ingests a mere two and a half servings of fruits and vegetables a day—a far cry from the recommended 5 to 7 servings.

Here is a listing of well-known phytonutrients and their benefits:

Chlorophyll

Source: green plants and other colored vegetables

Properties: antioxidant, contains vitamin K

Conditions: anemia, detoxification, burns and wounds, cancer prevention

Curcumin

Source: turmeric

Properties: anti-inflammatory, antioxidant

Conditions: arthritis, inflammatory bowel disease, cancer

Ellagic acid

Source: berries, grapes, apples, tea

Properties: detoxification

Conditions: cancer prevention

Flavoglycosides

Source: ginkgo, black tea

Properties: antioxidant, improves blood flow

Conditions: heart disease, kidney disease, varicose veins, depression, poor memory

Fructooligosaccharides (FOS)

Source: Jerusalem artichokes, chicory root, garlic, bananas

Properties: detoxification, increases beneficial bacteria

Conditions: digestive conditions such as irritable bowel syndrome, Crohn's disease, ulcerative colitis, yeast overgrowth, cancer, vaginitis

Gallic acid

Source: green tea, red wine
Properties: antioxidant, enhances immunity
Conditions: infections, heart disease

Glucosinolates

Source: cruciferous vegetables (broccoli, cauliflower, kale, Brussels sprouts)
Properties: detoxification, balances hormones
Conditions: cancer prevention, general detoxification

Indoles

Source: cruciferous vegetables (broccoli, cauliflower, kale, Brussels sprouts)
Properties: detoxification, balances hormones
Conditions: cancer prevention (especially hormone dependent such as breast and prostate)

Isoflavones

Source: soy
Properties: balances hormones
Conditions: PMS, menopause, cancer prevention

Isothiocyanates

Source: broccoli, cabbage, cauliflower, horseradish
Properties: detoxification
Conditions: cancer prevention

Lignans

Source: flaxseeds, walnuts
Properties: immune enhancement, balances hormones
Conditions: cancer prevention, cardiovascular disease prevention

Limonoids
Source: citrus fruits and peels
Properties: detoxification
Conditions: cancer prevention, cardiovascular disease prevention

Lycopene
Source: tomatoes, red grapefruit
Properties: antioxidant
Conditions: cancer prevention and treatment

Organosulfur compounds
Source: garlic, onions, chives
Properties: antioxidant, enhances immune system, detoxification
Conditions: cancer prevention, cardiovascular disease prevention, enhances immune system, general detoxification

Phenolic acids
Source: broccoli, berries, tomatoes, cabbage, whole grains
Properties: antioxidant
Conditions: cancer prevention

Sulforaphane
Source: cruciferous vegetables (broccoli, cauliflower, kale, Brussels sprouts)
Properties: detoxification, balances hormones
Conditions: cancer prevention

MIRACULOUS FIBER

Not only is fiber—which you can get only from plant foods—helpful for maintaining bowel regularity, but it can help with hormone balance, as well.

There are two main types of fiber: insoluble and soluble. Insoluble fiber (the type that doesn't dissolve in water) comes from leafy vegetables and wheat bran. It acts to bind excess estrogens, toxic xenoestrogens (and other hormones), as well as various toxins to waste matter as it passes through the digestive tract, thus preventing reabsorption into the bloodstream. Soluble fiber (the type that does dissolve in water) works to lower cholesterol and blood sugar. You get it from oat bran and beans.

Fiber also promotes the growth of beneficial bacteria such as *Lactobacillus acidophilus* in the digestive tract. These friendly bugs help metabolize hormones and prevent the overgrowth of unfriendly organisms such as *Candida*, a type of yeast. A high-fiber diet is also associated with a decreased risk of certain cancers.

The average American consumes somewhere between 11 to 20 grams of fiber daily. For optimal health, however, you should consume 40 to 50 grams daily. Following are some foods and their fiber content.

Serving size	Soluble Fiber (grams)	Insoluble Fiber (grams)	Total Fiber (grams)
FRUITS			
Apples, 1	0.4	2.6	3.0
Banana, 1	0.5	1.3	1.8
Blackberries, ½ cup	0.4	4.5	4.9
Blueberries, ½ cup	0.2	1.9	2.1
Grapefruit, ½	0.1	0.3	0.4
Grapes, 10	trace	0.5	0.5
Honeydew melon, ½ cup	0.1	0.4	0.5
Peach, 1	0.6	1.1	1.7
Raisins, ¼ cup	0.2	1.4	1.6
VEGETABLES			
Artichoke (fresh, cooked), 1 medium	3.5	2.9	6.4
Beans (black, dry cooked), ½ cup	0.1	2.7	2.8

Serving size	Soluble Fiber (grams)	Insoluble Fiber (grams)	Total Fiber (grams)
VEGETABLES *(Continued)*			
Broccoli, ½ cup	1.6	1.0	2.6
Brussels sprouts (frozen, cooked), ½ cup	0.4	2.8	3.2
Lettuce, ½ cup	0.2	0.3	0.5
Lentils (dry, cooked), ½ cup	0.1	2.8	2.9
Peas (green, canned, or frozen), ½ cup	0.3	2.8	3.1
Spinach, ½ cup cooked or canned, 2 cups raw	0.3	2.0	2.3
Vegetable soup (canned), 1 cup	0.6	1.6	2.1
GRAINS			
Bread, white or Italian, 1 slice	0.2	0.6	0.8
Bread, rye, 1 slice	0.2	0.5	0.7
Bread, whole wheat, 1 slice	0.3	2.2	2.5
Cereal, Total®, 1 cup	trace	0.8	0.9
Cereal, Rice Krispies®, 1 cup	0.1	0.4	0.5
Cereal, Special K® 1 cup	0.1	0.7	0.8
Cookies, oatmeal, 1 large	0.3	0.6	0.9
Cookies, plain sugar, 1	0.1	0.1	0.2
Crackers, Ritz®, 4	0.1	0.2	0.3
Muffin, blueberry, 1 small	0.2	0.6	0.8
Oats, whole, ½ cup	0.5	1.1	1.6
Pancakes, 2	0.2	0.7	0.9
Rice, medium grain, ½ cup	trace	0.3	0.4
NUTS			
Almonds, roasted, 22 whole	0.1	2.4	2.5
Peanuts, 30 to 40 whole	0.1	1.9	2.0
Walnuts, 14 halves	trace	1.0	1.1
LEGUMES			
Beans, black, ½ cup cooked	0.1	2.7	2.8
Lentils, ½ cup cooked	0.1	2.8	2.9

LOSE THE SIMPLE SUGARS

Simple sugars, such as those found in white bread, candy, soda, white rice, pasta, and crackers, are nutrient-poor foods that suppress the immune system. Much of the sugar people ingest is "hidden" in packaged foods under several different names such as fructose, maltodextrin, sucrose, dextrose, and others. Research has shown that the average American consumes 125 pounds of sugar a year. How much is that? Look at a 2-pound bag of sugar and then imagine 60 of them lined up in a row!

When a person consumes too many refined-sugar products, a condition known as insulin resistance can develop, which means that you may manufacture adequate insulin in your body, but you can't make full use of it. Refined sugar can also lead to another condition known as "Syndrome X," which comprises a cluster of symptoms that revolve around insulin resistance plus two of the following: high cholesterol, obesity (apple-shaped body due to excess fat around the belly or chest), high triglycerides, or high blood pressure. Researchers suspect that Syndrome X may be the penultimate step in the development of diabetes.

WHY WE EAT TOO MUCH SUGAR

Sugar is a carbohydrate, and carbohydrates can be very addicting. Why? Carbohydrates increase the body's store of the neurotransmitter known as serotonin, which gives us a feeling of well being. So the more sugar we eat, the more we artificially give ourselves a little boost of "happiness." Excessive, chronic ingestion of simple carbs, however, can lead to serotonin imbalance, which can cause lots of problems.

Pamela, for example, was a 49-year-old mother of two who was looking for a natural program to treat her "menopausal" symptoms, including lethargy and headaches. Pamela followed a diet that consisted, for the most part, of simple carbohydrates. For example, breakfast often included only a bagel and apple juice. Her favorite lunch was Alfredo pasta. Her natural program started with adding a quality protein source, such as fish, eggs, or soy to her meals, as well as steamed vegetables or a salad (and oatmeal for breakfast). Within a month, this simple dietary change made a dramatic improvement in Pamela's energy and headaches. The same dietary change probably would have helped her no matter what stage of life she had been in.

GOOD VS. BAD FATS

All fat is not created equal. Many different types of fats show up in our diet, some beneficial and some not so beneficial. It's important to know which are which because unhealthful fats can raise the risk for such serious illnesses and conditions as cancer, heart disease, and arthritis.

Among the harmful fats we consume are *saturated fats,* such as those found in red meat and dairy products, and *hydrogenated oils,* such as those found in margarine.

Among the beneficial fats are those known as *essential fatty acids,* which you must get from your diet, as your body cannot manufacture them. Essential fatty acids are critical to proper cell function; and, on a larger scale, they work to regulate hormone production and balance the immune and cardiovascular systems. They also play an important role in memory and mood, and are important to the proper functioning of many systems of the body.

Essential fatty acids are composed of three main groups:

- **Omega-3 fatty acids,** found in cold-water fish (salmon); flaxseed; walnuts; and supplements containing oils from fish (tuna, salmon, or cod), flaxseed, hemp, or perilla.

- **Omega-6 fatty acids** found in red meat; most vegetable oils such as safflower, sunflower; and walnuts.

- **Omega-9 fatty acids** found in olives and olive oil.

Please note that various foods contain different proportions of these essential fatty acids, and eating too much of one type and not enough of another can lead to problems. For example, vegetable oils are generally high in omega-6. Since vegetable oils are used in baked goods and fast foods, the average person gets an overabundance of omega-6 and not enough omega-3 and omega-9. This imbalance contributes to chronic disease and hormone imbalance. Thus, increasing your consumption of omega-3 and omega-9, and reducing omega-6 makes good sense.

QUALITY PROTEIN SOURCES

Although plant foods bring great benefits to your diet, quality protein foods are important as well. The amino acids that make up protein are required for the body's manufacture of hormones, enzymes, and many other life-sustaining substances.

Red meat products are high in protein, but they're also high in saturated fat, so eat them sparingly. Instead, focus on protein sources such as eggs, poultry, salmon, mackerel, trout, herring, and halibut. Of course, all animal products should be hormone- and antibiotic-free. Many vegetables, including legumes, corn, nuts, and seeds, also contain protein.

LIMIT THE FRIED FOODS

Frying foods—especially deep-frying—with some type of oil, butter, or margarine creates unnatural compounds such as trans-fatty acids, which can damage your immune system and cardiovascular system. You're much better off steaming, broiling, boiling, poaching, or lightly sautéing (with olive oil).

VARIETY

Every food has a different nutritional profile, so a varied diet will give you a wide spectrum of vitamins, nutrients, fiber, enzymes, and phytonutrients. On the other hand, when you constantly eat a monotonous diet consisting of only a few favorite foods, your chance of developing food sensitivities increases. So get out those healthy cookbooks and start experimenting with your meal plans.

MORE WATER, PLEASE

Because water should comprise over half of the weight of a healthy body, you need to maintain an adequate intake. If you don't, you won't function properly. In fact, that fatigue or those low-grade headaches you have been attributing to menopause may well be due to dehydration. Increased water intake is even more important for coffee lovers, as caffeine causes the body to lose water.

Make it a habit to drink purified water throughout the day—and don't wait until you're thirsty. Feeling thirsty means you're already quite low in water. Drink an 8-ounce glass of good old H_2O every two to three hours.

KEEP BALANCED WITH SOY

Unless you've been living in a cave somewhere, you have undoubtedly read or heard about the positive benefits of soy. Some scientists believe that Asian menopausal women experience fewer severe hot flashes and enjoy better bone health because of their high soy intake. Japanese women, for example, consume approximately 100 to 200 mg a day—far more than their American counterparts—and suffer far fewer menopausal symptoms.

Soy's phytoestrogens, such as genistein, daidzein, and glycetin, are thought to give the plant its hormone-balancing properties. One 12-week study of postmenopausal women found that consuming 60 grams of soy protein daily (containing 76 mg of isoflavones) resulted in a 45-percent reduction in daily hot flashes. Some women noticed their hot flashes diminishing within five days of adding soy to their diet.

Eating soy products can also help relieve vaginal dryness, improve bone density, and balance cholesterol levels.

Keep in mind that population studies have all been done on people who consume fermented soy foods such as miso, tofu, aburage tempeh, and others. Until isolated soy supplements are studied more in depth, it appears the fermented soy foods are the way to go.

Some of my patients cannot tolerate soy because they are sensitive to it. This problem usually presents itself in the form of gas and bloating. Supplemental enzymes taken with soy meals may help prevent this problem.

THE POWER OF FLAXSEEDS

Flaxseeds are a potent source of phytoestrogens. They contain phytonutrients known as lignans, which demonstrate phytoestrogenic (plant-source estrogen) activity. Flaxseeds are also an excellent source of omega-3 fatty acids and fiber, and have potent antioxidant activity. Flaxseeds help to reduce LDL cholesterol and increase beneficial HDL cholesterol, making them valuable for the cardiovascular system. Consuming a quarter cup of fresh, golden, ground-up flaxseeds on a daily basis is an excellent idea.

GREEN TEA INSTEAD OF COFFEE

You can get that caffeine boost in the morning without many of the disease-promoting properties of coffee. Your solution: green tea, which contains approximately half the amount of caffeine that coffee does, and an amino acid which relaxes the nerves. More important, it contains powerful antioxidants known as polyphenols, that are thought to play important roles in preventing cardiovascular disease and several types of cancer, including breast cancer. Green tea also contains vitamins C, D, K, and B2, as well as valuable minerals such as calcium, magnesium, chromium, manganese, iron, copper, zinc, molybdenum, selenium, and potassium.

Green tea enhances the liver's ability to detoxify the body and protects liver cells from damage. It also helps to improve digestive health by promoting the growth of friendly bacteria. Most Japanese and Chinese citizens drink green tea daily, and researchers feel this contributes greatly to the prevention of major chronic disease.

NOTE: To prevent disease and maintain wellness, drink two to three cups of green tea daily, preferably organic green tea, which is readily available. In addition, decaffeinated green tea is available for those sensitive to caffeine.

Coffee, on the other hand, severely depletes minerals, including calcium. Too much coffee (more than a cup or two daily) is associated with bone loss and osteoporosis. High amounts also contribute to anxiety, nervousness, and digestive upset. Finally, women who drink too much coffee can suffer from fatigue problems, as caffeine has been used as a stimulant and over time results in "adrenal fatigue."

GO ORGANIC

"Organic," as applied to foods, generally means they were produced without the aid of artificial chemicals. Why is this important? Pesticides, herbicides, and other synthetic insect repellants often present in nonorganic food can damage your immune and nervous systems. In addition, they mimic the effect of estrogen in the body and disrupt hormone balance. Plants, of course, aren't the only foods that can be nonorganic. Meat, poultry, dairy products, and eggs can contain hormones and antibiotics that you neither need nor want in your body. Fortunately, the demand for organic foods has increased so much that many grocery stores now carry these products.

EAT FRUIT INSTEAD OF CANDY

Want to satisfy your sweet craving? Sure, go ahead, but I recommend you focus on fruit instead of candy. Both are simple sugars and increase blood-sugar levels, but fruit offers nutritional advantages. Fruit contains vitamins, minerals, and enzymes, and, unlike candy—which is mostly sugar and coloring—it's packed with thousands of different phytonutrients.

For similar reasons, you should drink fruit and vegetable juices instead of soda and other soft drinks.

TRY STEVIA INSTEAD OF REFINED SUGAR OR ARTIFICIAL SWEETENERS

We all like the taste of sweetness. But we know that sugar, our favorite sweetener, is unhealthful for us. So what to do? Stevia, which is said to be sweeter than sugar, is a plant whose leaves have been used by South American people for hundreds of years. It does not have harmful effects on blood-sugar levels and is even safe for diabetics. It is available in powder and liquid concentrates. Use it in drinks or with cooking. You can find it in your local health food store and on the Internet.

EAT WHOLE-GRAIN PASTAS INSTEAD OF REFINED PASTAS

You probably love pasta if, like me, you're from an Italian heritage. However, many pastas are made out of refined flour products, which means the outer husk of the grain has been removed. It is this outer covering of the whole grain that contains fiber, phytonutrients, and valuable minerals such as magnesium. Fortunately, whole-grain pastas are readily available at supermarkets and health food stores.

EAT RICE, ALMOND, OR SOY MILK INSTEAD OF COW'S MILK

Have you looked at the choices of milk lately at your local supermarket or health food store? You'll find plenty of wonderful choices other than cow's milk. I frequently recommend calcium-enriched rice milk for my patients. It has as much calcium as cow's milk without the allergenic proteins that play havoc with so many people's immune systems, and it's lactose free.

Cow's milk, whether it is low fat or not, is a major source of lactose, a sugar that causes digestive upset (bloating, gas, diarrhea) in a great number of people. We know that 75 percent of adults have some degree of lactose intolerance. Those who are of northwest European descent are an exception, with an incidence of less than 20 percent. But 100 percent of Chinese and 75 percent of black Americans have lactase deficiency, as do a high percentage of those from Mediterranean descent.

So go with a substitute. If rice milk doesn't suit your taste, almond milk is another good choice, as is soy milk in moderate consumption.

DRINK PURIFIED WATER INSTEAD OF TAP WATER

You might think water from your kitchen tap is the purest thing you can put into your body, but that isn't necessarily so. Tap water is a source of chlorine that is associated with bladder cancer. Chlorine also destroys the friendly bacteria in your digestive tract. The media has reported in recent years that parasite infection is increasingly common in the water supply. In addition, toxic heavy metals, such as arsenic, lead, cadmium, and mercury, can also be found in the water supply.

Good clean water is necessary to maintain a healthy body. Bathe your cells in good water by investing in a quality filtration system for you and your family. Penta® water is an outstanding type of bottled water that I've frequently recommended to patients and use ourselves.

USE HERBAL SPICES INSTEAD OF SALT

Too much salt, especially in combination with a low intake of potassium, contributes to high blood pressure for some people. I also find salt leads to water retention and gives some women a bloated appearance.

Herbal spices, on the other hand, not only add flavor and zest to your meals, but in the long run can contribute to a healthy body. Turmeric, rosemary, and basil have been shown to have potent antioxidant activity. Oregano is a potent destroyer of viruses, bacteria, fungus, and parasites. Garlic helps to improve immunity, stop infections, and prevent heart disease as well as cancer.

Onions also fortify the immune system and contain valuable nutrients such as vitamin C and quercitin. Fennel not only adds flavor but prevents digestive upset, as does ginger.

DIGESTIVE HEALTH

The foods you eat influence your hormone balance, but so does the general health of your digestive tract. Having good bacteria such as *acidophilus* in your system plays an important role in hormone metabolism. However, many women suffer from *dysbiosis,* meaning an imbalance of the "good" and "bad" bacteria that inhabit the digestive, urinary, and vaginal areas. The use of antibiotics, anti-inflammatory medications, and chlorinated water destroy these helpful, friendly bacteria. In addition, refined sugar and alcohol feed "bad bugs" such as *Candida.* Chronic stress can also alter this important bacteria balance.

Fermented foods such as yogurt (with live cultures) and sauerkraut provide friendly bacteria. For more severe cases, probiotic supplements may be required.

USE OLIVE OIL INSTEAD
OF MARGARINE OR SHORTENING

Olive oil is rich in heart-healthy omega-9 fatty acids, which is why—as Greek and Italian population studies show—it protects against heart disease. Its use is also associated with a lower incidence of breast cancer.

Olive oil is much more stable than margarine or shortenings, which are more likely to go rancid. They're also high in the toxic trans-fatty acids, substances believed to contribute to heart disease, cancer, and many chronic diseases.

Add olive oil to your salads, and, if frying, use it instead of margarine. Extra-virgin olive oil is the type I recommend, especially if it's from an organic source.

6

$\mathcal{M}$ENOPAUSAL SUPPLEMENTS

$\mathcal{Y}$ou may have been taking supplements for most of your life, but your supplement needs are likely to change as menopause begins. This chapter is for all three mcnotypes, although the actual quantity and dosages of supplements are likely to differ for each type.

For example, calcium and the other bone-building minerals are critically important for menotype C's, who already may be afflicted with osteoporosis. Menotype B's and C's are also more likely to have a higher demand for the B vitamins, as their menopausal transition is more stressful, and stress "burns" up the m-B's much quicker.

Menotype B's and C's may have even higher supplement needs if they are on hormone therapy, as the liver requires a variety of nutrients to process hormones, whether natural or synthetic.

WHY THE NEED FOR SUPPLEMENTS?

Unfortunately, it can be nearly impossible to meet the daily recommended guidelines for vitamins and minerals by eating food alone. Refined and fast foods, depleted minerals in the soil, environmental toxins, lifestyle choices such as smoking and alcohol consumption, and stress increase the demand for certain nutrients. That's why it is important for women to understand the value of key supplements to meet their changing needs.

MULTIVITAMINS ARE A GOOD FIRST STEP

One way to ensure that a broad range of vitamins and minerals are amply supplied to the cells of your body is to take a multivitamin. A high-quality multivitamin really helps to prevent some chronic diseases. For example, some people have a genetic predisposition to build up a potentially toxic compound, homocysteine, in their bodies, which dramatically raises their risk for heart disease and stroke. Moderate doses of B vitamins such as B6, folic acid, and B12 prevent this from occurring. Minerals such as chromium and vanadium are needed for blood-sugar metabolism. The examples could go on, but you get the idea. All three menotypes would do well to use a multivitamin.

YOU DON'T NEED TO OVERDO THE IRON

One common mistake women make is that they take a multivitamin that contains iron, and in some cases a significant amount (15 mg or more).

Iron is a mineral with which you have to be careful. If you become too low in it, then symptoms such as easy bruising, fatigue, poor circulation, weakened immunity, spoon-shaped nails, and heavy or prolonged uterine bleeding can occur.

On the other hand, if you take iron and do not actually have an iron deficiency, then levels build up that can be hard on the liver. In addition, excess iron can promote oxidation and the formation of free radicals. Researchers feel this predisposes people to heart disease (due to oxidative damage to cholesterol) and possibly cancer (due to oxidative damage to cell DNA, which control cell division).

How do you know if you need to take a multivitamin containing iron? Some simple blood tests by your doctor are all that is needed. If you do not have iron-deficiency anemia, then you should not take any supplemental iron, even in a multivitamin. If your bloodwork shows that you are anemic, then it is prudent to take a multivitamin with iron or, in more serious cases of anemia, a separate iron supplement.

WHAT IS IN A GOOD MULTIVITAMIN?

A good multivitamin will contain a broad range of vitamins and minerals in adequate, proportional amounts. Following are the dosages to look for:

Vitamins

Vitamin A: 1,000–5,000 IU

Beta Carotene: 2,500 to 25,000 IU (mixed carotenoid complex is even better)

Vitamin D: 200–400 IU

Vitamin E: 400 IU (d-alpha tocopherol)

Vitamin K: 200–500 mcg (not allowed in Canadian formulations)

Vitamin C: 100–1,000 mg

Vitamin B1(thiamin): 10–100 mg

Vitamin B2 (riboflavin): 10–50 mg

Vitamin B3 (niacin): 10–100 mg

Niacinamide: 10–50 mg

Vitamin B5 (pantothenic acid): 25–100 mg

Vitamin B6 (pyridoxine): 25–100 mg

Folic Acid: 400–800 mcg

Vitamin B12: 400–800 mcg

Choline: 10–100 mg

Inositol: 10–100 mg

Minerals

Calcium: 250–1,000 mg

Magnesium: 250–500 mg

Chromium: 200–400 mcg

Copper: 1–2 mg

Manganese: 5–15 mg

Molybdenum: 10–25 mcg

Selenium: 200 mcg

Boron: 1–3 mg (not allowed in Canadian formulations)

Silica: 1–20 mg

Vanadium: 50–100 mcg

Zinc: 15–30 mg

Absorption

I do prefer capsules and powders over whole tablets for improved absorption, although some tablets do absorb well (depending on the brand). Most high-potency multivitamins require two to six capsules, or two or more tablets daily.

In addition to the form of the multivitamin itself, good digestive function is important for efficient absorption. It is well established that adequate stomach acid is required for many minerals to be absorbed. However, it is very common for menopausal and postmenopausal women to have low stomach acid.

Betaine hydrochloride tablets taken with meals (when you also take the multivitamin) or herbal digestive tonics, such as Gentian and Ginger Root, can help stimulate production of stomach acid.

Consistency

Buying high-quality multivitamins, of course, is not helpful if they sit on the shelf of your medicine cabinet or if you take them only when the mood strikes you. You need to take supplements consistently so that your cells can maintain levels adequate to function properly.

If you miss a day or two here and there, however, don't worry, don't give up, and don't take any extra amounts to make up for the missed doses. The damaging effects of nutritional deficiencies do not occur overnight, but rather, over months and years of inadequate intake. Just pick up where you left off, and go on taking your multivitamin as usual.

PINPOINTING AREAS OF DEFICIENCY

Even though a multivitamin gives you a wide range of nutrients, you may still experience deficiencies that result from your genetics, diet, environmental exposure, state of health, or medications you are taking.

How do you know if you're deficient? One option is to do specialized lab testing. Blood and urine tests are available to measure several different vitamins and minerals. Unfortunately, they tend to be quite expensive, but if you can afford them and work with a holistic doctor who can interpret the results, they can be very helpful. Labs that perform these specialized tests are included in the Resources at the end of this book.

NOTE: Hair analysis can be used to assess certain minerals. However, it is accurate for only a limited number of minerals and is of no value for vitamins. Labs that specialize in hair analysis are included in the Resources.

SUPPLEMENTS YOU MAY NEED

A more practical method for most women to assess vitamin and mineral needs is to assess their own signs, symptoms, and health conditions.

Following are some of the vitamins and minerals for which many of my female patients need to do extra supplementation. Do you need to take all of the vitamins and minerals listed here? No, but if you have symptoms or conditions that are "indicators" for any particular vitamin or mineral, then supplementation may be required.

It is always recommended that you work with a knowledgeable health practitioner when deciding on a supplement program. The following information is intended to point you in the right direction.

Calcium

We all know that calcium is vitally important for bone health, yet most women do not take in enough on a daily basis to protect against the ravages of osteoporosis. ***Dosage:*** The National Academy of Sciences recommends adults 19 to 50 years old consume 1,000 mg and those 51 years or older consume 1,200 mg daily.

Calcium has many more benefits than simply supporting bone health. It helps relax the nervous system and muscles, which is especially beneficial for people suffering from muscle cramps and spasms. Supplementation helps many women sleep better. It has also been shown effective for the treatment of PMS, and can help lower blood pressure. Studies are also showing that it protects against colon cancer and high cholesterol levels.

Women of all ages would be wise to supplement with 500 mg (minimum) to 1,000 mg (optimum) of calcium daily. This includes the amount in your multivitamin. Women with osteoporosis should try supplementing with 1,000 to 1,200 mg daily.

The form of calcium is very important as different forms absorb better than others. I recommend calcium citrate or citrate-malate because of all the positive studies done on these forms.

Medications known to deplete calcium
caffeine
prednisone
many different antibiotics
Losartan® (hypertension medication)
thiazide diuretics

NOTE: Persons with hyperparathyroidism and kidney disease should not supplement calcium unless under a doctor's supervision.

Calcium interferes with iron and zinc absorption. If high levels of these minerals are required, they should be taken at least four hours before or after you take your calcium.

Indicators for calcium

Muscle aches and cramps	Osteoporosis
Insomnia	Angina
Joint pain	Diabetes
High blood pressure	Migraines

Magnesium

This mineral is required for several hundred enzymatic reactions in your cells every second, including energy production and detoxification. Magnesium is the second most abundant mineral in the cells (potassium is first). It is also very important for bone health.

An average daily dose is 500 mg, including what is in your multivitamin. *50 mg*

Medications known to deplete magnesium

digoxin

corticosteroids

birth-control pills

theophylline

warfarin

NOTE: Women with kidney disease should not supplement with magnesium unless instructed to do so by a physician. It should not be taken at the same time as the drugs Fosamax®, cimetidine, ranitidine, and tetracycline; instead, take it a few hours later.

Indicators for magnesium

Muscle weakness, spasms, cramps, and soreness

Fatigue

Insomnia

Irritability

Anxiety

Heart arrhythmias and heart disease

Osteoporosis

Fibromyalgia

Sweet cravings

Hypertension

Kidney stones

Vitamin E (d-alpha tocopherol)

The Nurses' Health Study, which involved 87,000 women, found that those who took vitamin E for two years or more had a 41-percent reduction in their risk for heart disease. Given that heart disease is the number-one killer of women, it makes sense to boost the levels of this wondrous antioxidant. Some women also find it effective for hot flashes and breast tenderness related to fibrocystic breast syndrome.

An average daily dose of vitamin E is between 400 to 800 IU. For the relief of hot flashes or breast tenderness, up to 1,200 IU may be required.

Always purchase the natural form, which is d-alpha tocopherol as opposed to the synthetic version, which is d'l-alpha tocopherol. Although it costs more, the natural form is approximately three times more bioavailable to the body's tissues. Optimally, a "mixed" vitamin E is optimal, which contains a blend of all the naturally occuring tocopherols.

Tocotrienols are also a part of the vitamin E family, and are found in foods such as cereal bran, rice bran, wheat bran, and oat bran. Research is showing that the tocotrienols help to lower cholesterol and treat hardening of the arteries.

An average daily dosage for tocotrienols for a healthy person ranges from 20 to 80 mg. Those with high cholesterol may need tocotrienol dosages as high as 400 mg (tocotrienols can be purchased as a separate supplement for people needing very high dosages). Work with a nutrition-oriented doctor when using the tocotrienols for these conditions.

NOTE: If you are on blood-thinning medications, consult with your doctor first before supplementing vitamin E.

Medications known to deplete vitamin E

certain chemotherapy drugs

Indicators for vitamin E

Heart disease	Cancer prevention
Muscle weakness	Diabetes
Hot flashes	Acne
Breast tenderness	Angina
Arthritis	

SHE TRIED IT

Penny, a 49-year-old nurse, had noticed substantial improvement of her hot flashes using a menopause herbal supplement that contained Black Cohosh. She was also taking a soy supplement. However, she felt that her hot flashes were still too strong and that her fibrocystic breast syndrome was flaring up. Since she was a menotype B, we had her supplement 1,200 IU of vitamin E—which made the difference Penny needed within three weeks of use.

Vitamin C

Vitamin C does more than help ward off the common cold. This water-soluble antioxidant also helps protect against cell damage, maintain skin integrity through the formation of the skin protein collagen, produce stress-fighting hormones, support immune function, and protect against heart disease and cancer.

A recent study reported in the *Lancet* medical journal found a small increase in vitamin C intake could produce a substantial reduction in cardiovascular mortality. Researchers measured plasma ascorbic acid concentrations in 19,496 men and women aged 45–79 years and followed them for four years. An increase in plasma ascorbic acid concentration was strongly and independently associated with a reduction in premature mortality from all causes, cardiovascular disease, and heart disease. Vitamin C was also associated with a decreased risk of death related to cancer in men.

Obviously, it's a good idea to consume fruits and vegetables high in vitamin C such as citrus fruits, tomatoes, peppers, dark-green leafy vegetables, broccoli, kale, strawberries, and potatoes.

Many people also benefit from vitamin C supplementation. This is particularly true of people with arthritis, asthma, allergies, diabetes, gingivitis, cataracts, and those needing immune support.

An average daily dosage is 500 to 1,000 mg of supplemental vitamin C. If you take too much, then you may experience diarrhea, which will go away when you cut down the dose. People with infections, cancer, and other chronic diseases may require substantially higher dosages. Since it is a water-soluble vitamin, it is best taken in divided doses throughout the day. Some people cannot tolerate regular vitamin C as it upsets their stomach or causes other reactions. Ester-C® or calcium ascorbate are buffered and therefore better tolerated.

Medications known to deplete vitamin C

corticosteroids

certain chemotherapy drugs

indomethacin

tetracycline

Indicators for vitamin C

Easy bruising

Bleeding gums

Slow wound healing

Reoccurring infections

Cancer prevention

Cardiovascular disease prevention

Diabetes

B vitamins

High stress, the use of hormones, and too many refined grains in the diet are three key reasons why many menopausal patients need extra B vitamins. Physical and mental stresses have been shown to "burn" up B vitamins. Hormones such as Premarin® may deplete the body of B6 and other nutrients, and refined grain products are poor sources of B vitamins.

Lifestyle choices such as excessive alcohol consumption, smoking, and high caffeine intake can also lead to the loss of B vitamins.

There are several different B vitamins, each of which has a different function. As a group, they help to produce energy and combat the effects of stress.

Here's what they do individually:

- **Vitamin B1 (thiamine)** deficiency can impair memory and mood. This is seen more commonly in alcoholics.

- **Vitamin B2 (riboflavin)** is helpful for some people, when used at a dosage of 400 mg daily, for the prevention of chronic migraine headaches.

- **Vitamin B3 (niacin)** works to combat high cholesterol levels when used at dosages of 1,500 mg or higher.

- **Vitamin B5 (pantothenic acid)** is required to produce adrenal hormones.

- **Vitamin B6 (pyridoxine)** works to reduce homocysteine, a substance implicated in heart disease.

- **Folic acid** is needed for proper cell division. A deficiency can result in fatigue, poor memory, neuropathy, depression, and several other problems.

- **Vitamin B12** is also required for cell division and energy production. A deficiency can result in fatigue, poor memory, neuropathy, depression, and other problems.

If you need extra supplementation, take a 50-mg B-complex in addition to your multivitamin (which contains a spectrum of B vitamins). In certain cases, individual B vitamins may need to be taken, such as B6 for carpal tunnel syndrome or B3 for high cholesterol. I certainly recommend an extra B-complex for menotype C's who are using hormone replacement, especially synthetic hormones such as Premarin®.

Medications known to deplete B vitamins

birth-control pill
Premarin®
seizure medications
ulcer drugs
steroid medications

Indicators for B vitamins

Fatigue
Mood swings

Elevated cholesterol and cardiovascular markers

Water retention

Chronic cold sores and canker sores

Super antioxidants

Antioxidants are proving quite valuable in the prevention of many serious illnesses such as cancer and heart disease. Some researchers even claim that antioxidants can slow down the aging process. Essentially, they prevent cell DNA from becoming damaged. They do this by neutralizing free radicals, which are unstable molecules that may become damaging to the tissues and organs of the body.

Illnesses such as arthritis and cataracts may be slowed with adequate amounts of antioxidants. Those who expose themselves to too much sun or who smoke require extra antioxidant protection, as well. People who are very physically active generate more free radicals and can benefit from antioxidants.

People with high cholesterol can also benefit from antioxidants. Interestingly, high cholesterol in the bloodstream remains harmless until it becomes oxidized. Guess what shields against the oxidation of cholesterol? Yes, antioxidants.

There is a long list of antioxidants. It is impractical to purchase all of them individually, although it makes sense to do so with some such as vitamin C, E, and CoQ10. Generally, you'll want to use an antioxidant complex supplement, many of which are readily available at your health food store and on the Internet. Make sure you get a full spectrum of the antioxidants, instead of super-high levels of just one or two.

Common antioxidants

Vitamin A (*Dosage:* 2,500–5,000 IU)

Vitamin C (*Dosage:* 500–1,000 mg)

Vitamin E (*Dosage:* 400–800 IU)

Selenium (*Dosage:* 200–400 mcg)

Carotenoids (*Dosage:* mixed carotenoid complex [25 mg])

Lipoic Acid (*Dosage:* 50–100 mg)

Grape Seed Extract or Pycnogenol (*Dosage:* 50–100 mg)

Coenzyme Q10 (*Dosage:* 30–50 mg)

Minerals for Blood-Sugar Balancing

Your blood-sugar level has a profound effect on the way you feel. If you have problems with blood sugar, such as hypoglycemia or diabetes, the following minerals can be helpful when used along with a good diet and exercise. Essentially, they help with the proper transport and metabolism of glucose within cells.

NOTE: If you are on diabetic medication, then consult with your doctor before using these supplements, as your medication may need to be lowered over time.

Chromium (*Dosage:* 200–600 mcg daily)

Vanadium (*Dosage:* 300 mg of vanadyl sulfate or 100 mcg of elemental vanadium)

Alpha Lipoic Acid (*Dosage:* 200 600 mg daily)

Essential Fatty Acids

Essential fatty acids are so named because your body cannot manufacture them, and you require them to live. The vast majority of women I see have some degree of essential-fatty-acid-deficiency. Fast foods and the creation of "synthetic fats" by the food industry have led to a severe problem with essential-fatty-acid imbalance. The most common symptoms include dry skin, brittle hair and nails, poor circulation, arthritis, and poor memory. In addition, persons deficient in the omega-3 fatty acids found in such foods as salmon and flaxseeds are at greater risk for heart disease.

With regard to supplements, the two main sources are fish oils (such as salmon oil) and flaxseed oil. Both are good sources of heart-healthy and immune-supportive omega-3 fatty acids. However, for inflammatory conditions, you should take fish oil extract, as most of the studies have been done with this form.

Oil blends are also a good idea and may include a source of essential fatty acid GLA (gamma linolenic acid), which is usually derived from evening primrose or borage oil. I do not advocate taking either of these two oils by themselves though, as they are sources of omega-6 fatty acids (which most people get too much of as it is). GLA can be very helpful for chronic breast tenderness.

Flaxseed oil (*Dosage:* 1–2 tablespoons daily)

Fish oil (*Dosage:* 1,000–6,000 mg daily)

Oil blend (*Dosage:* as directed on container)

Digestive Enzymes

It seems as if almost every patient I talk to has one digestive problem or another, including gas, bloating, and constipation. Good digestion is an absolute must for good health.

Digestive enzymes can help with these problems. These are enzymes that, when taken with meals, help to break down food more efficiently. Three main types of enzymes are commercially available: animal, plant, and microbial-derived.

I prefer microbial-derived enzymes, which are usually grown on the fungus *Aspergillus oryzae* and then go through an intensive purification process. You can find them in health food stores and some pharmacies. Take two capsules with each meal.

NOTE: Digestive enzymes should not be used by persons with gastritis or ulcers.

Probiotics

Antibiotics have saved many lives, but indiscriminate use has come with a cost. Broad-spectrum antibiotics destroy beneficial as well as harmful bacteria, particularly in your digestive, respiratory, and urinary tract. Chlorinated water, anti-inflammatory medicines, and stress also deplete the body's supply of friendly microbes.

These good bacteria or "flora" serve many functions, such as preventing harmful bacteria and other microbes from overgrowing. They also help synthesize certain vitamins, including vitamin K and several B vitamins.

With regard to women's health, they help metabolize estrogen so that toxic metabolites (byproducts) do not accumulate in the body. They also prevent chronic vaginal yeast infections.

Probiotics are products that contain the beneficial bacteria such as *Lactobacillus acidophilus,* bifidus, and others. Look for refrigerated formulas that contain at least two billion organisms per daily serving. Also, products are available that contain a substance called FOS (fructooligosaccharides) that supports the selective growth of *Lactobacillus acidophilus* and bifidobacteria. Take between meals for a minimum of two months. By the way, you need not worry about overdoing probiotics. The normal, healthy human body carries over four pounds of friendly flora!

LOOKING FOR RELIABLE BRANDS

When it comes to nutritional supplements, the old advice of "Buyer beware" makes a lot of sense. Not all supplement brands are of the same quality, potency, and purity. As in many industries, some supplement companies have exceptionally high standards and make quality products; others don't. How can this be? Currently, the supplement industry is self-regulated in the United States. In other words, manufacturers and distributors are on the honor system. As you might expect, some people cut corners to reduce cost when making a product. Some products don't even meet the claims on their own labels.

The situation may soon change. Right now the health food industry is working on developing new standards and quality-control procedures for everyone to follow. Meanwhile, there are some excellent supplement brands that are readily available to you through health food stores, pharmacies, the Internet, and direct mail. I recommend that you consult with your local naturopathic doctor, holistic medical doctor, nutritionist, or other natural healthcare practitioner for recommendations concerning quality brands. Experienced health food store employees can also help provide information on products and quality brands.

DRUG-INDUCED
NUTRITIONAL DEFICIENCIES

More physicians are becoming aware of the fact that pharmaceuticals have the potential to induce one or more nutritional deficiencies. Following are common pharmaceuticals and the nutrients in which they are known to induce deficiencies.

Premarin® and Provera®
- Vitamin B6
- Zinc
- Magnesium

Mevacor®
- Coenzyme Q10

Zantac®
- Vitamin B12

Aspirin
- Vitamin C

Oral Contraceptives
- Folic acid
- Magnesium
- Vitamins B1, B2, B3, B6, B12
- Vitamin C

Tricyclic Antidepressants and Beta Blockers
- CoQ10

7

$\mathcal{H}$OMEOPATHY

$\mathcal{H}$omeopathy can be just what the doctor ordered for menotypes A and B. This form of nontoxic, natural medicine works to alleviate common menopausal symptoms in the gentlest way possible. As a matter of fact, in the vast majority of cases, homeopathy will be the only therapy you need for the mild hot flash or occasional mood swing that a menotype A experiences.

For the menotype B who experiences troublesome hot flashes or lowered libido, homeopathy can seem miraculous, and it can help relieve a menoptype C of symptoms such as fatigue, depression, insomnia, or arthritis, though she will still require hormone therapy as her primary treatment.

LIKE CURES LIKE

You have probably heard the term "homeopathy" and may even have seen homeopathic "remedies" in your local health food store or pharmacy, but how this treatment differs from other types of holistic or natural healing may remain a mystery for you.

Homeopathy developed from the idea that a substance that causes particular symptoms in a healthy person can cure or improve those same symptoms in someone who is ill. As an example, let's take the homeopathic remedy Belladonna. If you were to ingest the Belladonna plant (which is not recommended as it can be quite toxic), you would probably react first by flushing deeply, especially in the face, and then sweating profusely. But in a menopausal woman suffering from hot flashes—essentially the same symptoms—we can use a homeopathic preparation of Belladonna, diluted until it's no longer toxic, as a treatment.

WHAT THE REST OF THE WORLD KNOWS THAT WE DON'T

Homeopathy is just beginning to enjoy resurgence in popularity among healthcare professionals and the public in North America, but it has long been used by the medical establishments in other countries. For example, in Germany, approximately 40 percent of all medical doctors prescribe homeopathic remedies or refer to practitioners that do. According to Dana Ullman, coauthor of *Everybody's Guide to Homeopathic Medicines,* over 70,000 registered homeopaths practice in India. Another country with a strong homeopathic following is Britain, which is home to the Royal London Homeopathic Hospital. In France, more than 6,000 physicians practice homeopathy and over 18,000 pharmacies sell homeopathic remedies. You get the picture: Homeopathy is not some new fad practiced by a handful of "country doctors." Scientific studies have been done on specific homeopathic medicines. As you might expect, some results are positive and some are not, as is always the case when substances are tested for their effectiveness.

YOU ARE NOT ALONE

In the United States, many people have long held the idea that using homeopathic remedies is a little . . . well . . . eccentric. But things are changing. Today, well-known celebrities such as Jane Seymour and Lindsey Wagner strongly endorse homeopathic medicine and testify to the benefits homeopathy has given to them and their families. If the experience of Hollywood's elite doesn't convince you, then consider this: The Royal Family in England has been under homeopathic care since 1930.

HOW TO PICK THE RIGHT HOMEOPATHIC REMEDY

There are two ways to choose a homeopathic remedy. One is to pick the remedy that best matches your symptoms. This is the preferred method and the one most homeopathic practitioners use.

However, vague symptoms can cloud the situation, especially for the lay person. In this case, your best option might be to purchase a combination remedy. By the term combination I am referring to a homeopathic formula containing the most common remedies (usually five or more) for whatever general condition or ailment you wish to treat.

Several homeopathic brands carry "Menopause" formulas, which contain remedies for the most common symptoms women experience during their transition. If your symptoms are unusual, however, you may need to find out which specific remedy will work for you. Consulting with a homeopathic practitioner may be your best bet. To find one where you live, I have provided the names of some reputable referral agencies in the Resources section of this book.

WHAT POTENCY TO USE

Potency refers to the strength of a remedy. The number behind the name of the homeopathic indicates the dilution and strength of the medicine. The higher the number, the stronger the action of the remedy. For example, 30C is stronger than 12C, and 12X is stronger than 6X.

Here are the two common scales of homeopathy available in the marketplace:

"X": X stands for a 1-in-9 dilution. So 1X is equal to 1 part of the original substance diluted in 9 parts of solution.

"C": C stands for a 1-in-99 dilution. Thus, 1C is equal to 1 part of the original substance in 99 parts of solution. Stores often carry 30C potencies for many of the remedies.

HOW TO USE HOMEOPATHICS

If you find a homeopathic remedy that fits your symptoms, then by all means try it and see if it makes a difference. Please note that you need not have all the symptoms listed in the following remedies. If you see two or three symptoms that match yours, then that remedy is worth trying.

What you will generally find with homeopathic remedies is that they either are very helpful or they do nothing at all. In some cases, improvement may follow an initial aggravation of symptoms. I generally recommend two pellets of a 30C potency (as this is the potency most commonly available) be taken twice daily. Menopausal symptoms will usually improve within seven days. If there is no improvement within that time, try another remedy or consult with a homeopathic practitioner. After you first notice improvement, stop taking the remedy unless symptoms begin to return, in which case repeat the remedy for a couple of days.

If you're using an "X" potency (6X, 12X), take it three times daily.

COMMON MENOPAUSAL REMEDIES

Following are the "Big 7," that is, the seven most common remedies for perimenopause and menopause.

Belladonna

This remedy is useful for "throbbing" hot flashes that cause a red facial flush along with or followed by sweating. Heart palpitations and restlessness are also characteristic symptoms. Belladonna can also help relieve right-sided, throbbing headaches that began with the menopausal change.

Lachesis Mutas

This remedy can be used to treat hot flashes that are quite strong. It is one of the best menopausal remedies for treating heart palpitations that get worse when you're lying on your left side. It can also alleviate heavy menstrual flow that displays purplish clots. It is an important remedy for women who undergo intense emotions as they pass into menopause, including jealousy, anger, and suspiciousness that makes the affected woman feel like lashing out at someone. One sign that this remedy will work for you: You have an extremely high sex drive during the transition.

SHE TRIED IT

Toni had tried several natural products and treatments for relief of her hot flashes, among them herbs, acupuncture, and synthetic hormones, but she obtained only mild relief. Since entering menopause, her blood pressure had become moderately elevated as well. Based on her symptoms, I prescribed Belladonna for her. She soon experienced a decrease in the intensity of her hot flashes as well as an average lowering of 15 points in her blood pressure. As treatment went on, the combination of Belladonna and natural progesterone did the trick for Toni, who was a menotype B.

SHE TRIED IT

Wilma came to our clinic after hearing one of my lectures on natural approaches to menopause. Among her biggest concerns were her feelings of rage with her kids at home and with her employees at work. She was sure that hormone imbalance had a lot to do with how she felt, since she could find no other reason for her rages. Wilma was also experiencing strong hot flashes and insomnia. Lachesis Mutas was prescribed with good results. Over the first two weeks, Wilma noticed a decrease in the intensity and frequency of her hot flashes. With time, she also began to feel more "cheery and warm." People were commenting on how much more "peaceful" she was and asked what type of "hormones" she was taking. Wilma's experience demonstrates just how powerful homeopathy can be.

Natrum Muriaticum

While this remedy can help hot flashes and vaginal dryness, it is more known for treating depression that occurs during menopause. A woman who needs this remedy often wants to be alone. She feels like crying easily, yet does not want people to see her crying or try to comfort her. It is an effective treatment for insomnia that began along with depression during perimenopause. It is one of the most common remedies for migraine headaches, especially headaches brought on by being out in the sun. One peculiar sign that tells you this is the right remedy for you: You experience a strong craving for salt.

SHE TRIED IT

Pauline came to my office for treatment of her depression. After taking her history, it became clear that her problem began when she had first become perimenopausal almost two years ago. Although her medical doctor had recommended hormone replacement and Prozac®, Pauline refused. She did have a strong craving for salty foods and described how she loaded salt onto whatever she ate. Natrum Muriaticum was prescribed and a lifting of her depression resulted over the following three months. Pauline continues on homeopathic treatment and has been able to resume a normal social life.

SHE TRIED IT

Both of Celine's ovaries had been removed due to ovarian cancer when she was 46. Due to the type of cancer she'd had, her doctor advised that she not use any type of hormones. However, severe hot flashes became a problem soon after the surgery. Oophorinum was prescribed and provided dramatic relief of the hot flashes within five days of use. Now, two years later, Celine continues to use this remedy, but only if she feels her symptoms returning.

Oophorinum (Ovary Extract)

This homeopathic preparation of the ovary is a remedy specific for menotype-C women. It is used for hot flashes and other menopausal symptoms caused by surgical removal of the ovaries.

Pulsatilla

The woman requiring this remedy usually experiences hot flashes when in a warm environment. The dead-giveaway sign that you need this remedy is general weepiness. Unlike Natrum Muriaticum, the affected woman can cry in front of others, and she desires to have company and to be consoled. Women who respond well to Pulsatilla often display a strong craving for chocolate, sweets, and pastries.

SHE TRIED IT

Kara suspected that perimenopause was to blame when her cycle became very irregular and her emotions unstable. She described how she would cry all the time, often for no apparent reason. This emotional distress would disappear temporarily when she ate chocolate. After taking Pulsatilla for three weeks, however, Kara felt her emotions "smooth out." Although she still felt weepy at times, her emotions were more controllable and not so "overly dramatic" as they had been. Her menstrual flow also lightened.

Sepia

This is among the most common remedies women use during menopause. It treats hot flashes accompanied by profuse sweating. It can also alleviate vaginal dryness, uterine prolapse, and urinary incontinence, and can improve weak or irregular menstrual flow that started with perimenopause. Women who fit the Sepia picture usually have a low libido or an outright aversion to sex, even if they're happily married. They generally crave sweets, especially chocolate, as well as vinegar and salty foods. They often describe themselves (or appear) "burned out" from the depression and irritability that began with the change of life, and they prefer being alone.

SHE TRIED IT

"He is a good man but I just start yelling at him for the littlest things," exclaimed Beth as she described how she had been feeling toward her husband for the past four months. Beth was also experiencing severe hot flashes during menopause, and when asked about her libido, she bluntly commented, "I might as well be a nun, which doesn't make my husband too happy." Before trying hormones, Beth was given Sepia, which turned out to work wonders for her. The hot flashes improved significantly within the first four weeks and her irritability and temper calmed down greatly. It took another three months before her libido started to come back.

Sulphur

This remedy is good for treating intense hot flashes (described as burning) and night sweats. The woman who responds well to sulphur feels hot all the time and perspires easily. She often feels an acute thirst for cold drinks. Her head is very hot, and her hands and feet burn. She throws her bed covers off at night or sticks her feet and hands out of the covers because she feels too warm.

SHE TRIED IT

"I used to be chilly all the time, now I am like a furnace 24 hours a day," stated Sheila. The only thing that provided Sheila some temporary relief was ice cold drinks. She was very restless at night, tossing and turning. She slept without wearing any clothes because her night sweats were so bad. She fit the menotype-B profile, so I decided to start her on homeopathic Sulphur. Fortunately, the remedy helped to "cool" her down, and her menopausal experience became much more pleasant.

8

&XERCISE

Motivation is an important factor in any exercise program, but it can be a difficult challenge if you're coping with hot flashes or depression. So it should come as no surprise that menotype C's often find it difficult to start exercising. If the menotype C can make it through the first two weeks of an exercise program, however, the benefits and feeling of renewed vitality will start to become evident. Often, C's report great improvements in circulation, depression, and insomnia, and, for many, regular exercise is absolutely necessary to regain bone density and reverse the start of cardiovascular disease.

Menotype A's should have no problem at all getting into the "swing" of an exercise program. A's do not have the distracting menopausal symptoms of the other types. However, they may still find it a challenge to remain consistent in their workout routine.

Menotype B's may find it harder to get going, but the effort is well worth it. Regular exercise is one of the keys to preventing the need for hormones or medications during menopause, and it "smoothes out" depression, anxiety, and the general effects of stress.

EXERCISE AND MENOPAUSE

Exercise is good for everyone, but it has special benefits for women in perimenopause and menopause. Here are some of them.

TAME HOT FLASHES. Exercise can be a powerful tool in reducing the intensity of hot flashes. Although there are conflicting studies in this area, its value is obvious in many of my patients. One Swedish study of almost 800 women found that only 5 percent of highly physically active women experienced severe hot flashes, as compared with 14 to 16 percent of women who had little or no weekly exercise. This information is particularly important for menotypes B and C.

REDUCE YOUR RISK OF HEART DISEASE AND STROKE. Want a real good reason to exercise? Each year in the United States, 500,000 women experience heart attacks, but regular exercise can *cut your risk* of a heart attack by a third to a half. Consistent physical activity has been shown to lower high blood pressure, support balanced cholesterol levels, and improve sluggish circulation. Inactivity, on the other hand, is the most prevalent risk factor for heart disease. A sedentary lifestyle is more predictive of heart disease than diet, smoking, or alcohol intake.

Edward Lakatta, M.D., chief of the Laboratory of Cardiovascular Science at the National Institute on Aging, says, ". . . [A]erobic exercise conditioning can offset normal aging of the heart by making it a better pump, even for those who begin later in life. . . . [Y]ou don't lose the ability to get into better condition."

Even so simple an exercise as brisk walking can substantially reduce your risk for cardiovascular disease and stroke. The Nurses' Health Study, which involved 72,488 female nurses between the ages of 40 and 65, demonstrated that brisk walking, or striding, seems to lower a woman's risk of stroke, compared with average or casual pace of walking.

IMPROVE YOUR MOOD. Exercise has a positive effect on the balance of brain chemicals that are responsible for mood and behavior. In my own practice, I have found exercise to be quite helpful in reducing depression and anxiety for women going through perimenopause and menopause.

Research on the subject seems to show similar results. Two studies by Australian scientists looked at the impact of exercise on menopausal symptoms.

The first study showed that the exercisers' moods remained significantly more positive than the sedentary women's moods, regardless of the menopausal state. Exercisers also had fewer physical symptoms and memory-concentration difficulties.

The second study focused on the immediate effects of aerobic exercise. The researchers found substantial improvements in mood and reductions in physical symptoms following aerobic classes. The study authors concluded, "Exercise may assist in the alleviation of some menopausal symptoms."

REDUCE YOUR RISK OF DIABETES. Diabetes is a serious disease whose incidence is increasing among all age groups, but people who exercise regularly are less likely to develop adult-onset diabetes. Aerobic activity promotes the body's ability to control blood-glucose levels by increasing insulin sensitivity and reducing body fat. Exercise is an undisputed weapon in the prevention and treatment of diabetes.

IMPROVE BONE DENSITY. Exercise is critical to good bone density and the prevention and treatment of osteoporosis. This debilitating condition is responsible for chronic pain, spine problems, and bone fractures for millions of senior citizens. However, bone loss is preventable and, to some extent, reversible. How? Active people lose bone mass more slowly.

Studies have shown that consistent weight-bearing exercise increases bone density. Muscle contraction exerts pressure on the bones, thereby stimulating bone-density growth. Good forms of weight-bearing exercise include walking, jogging, weight-lifting, and racquet sports. Interestingly, studies have also indicated that certain nonweight-bearing exercises, such as swimming, also increase bone density.

Of course, any type of exercise that improves coordination and flexibility can reduce the risk of a fall and thus a fracture. This is very important for all women, particularly menotype C's.

IMPROVE YOUR QUALITY OF SLEEP. Sleeplessness is another unfortunate but reversible symptom of menopause. Some medications promote sleep but may lead to grogginess and addiction. Exercise offers a natural alternative, and the only side effects are reduced body fat, stronger bones, a clearer head, pain relief, and a reduced risk of heart disease and type 2 diabetes.

RELIEVE PAIN. As you read in Chapter 1, arthritis often becomes a problem during menopause. Exercise is key in helping to cope with the pain of the many different types of arthritis, especially the most common type, osteoarthritis, which is a gradual degeneration of the joints. When you exercise, your body releases natural pain-relieving chemicals called endorphins, as well as other natural anti-inflammatory chemicals. Physical activity also improves circulation through the joints, which aids in healing and prevents tissue breakdown.

Arthritis isn't the only cause of chronic pain during menopause. Low back pain is common as well. One study investigated the effect of exercise on adults with low back pain. The 187 participants either underwent usual primary care management, or attended exercise classes that included strengthening, stretching, and relaxation exercises. After one year, the patients who exercised showed significantly greater improvement of their back pain. They also reported only 378 days off work, as compared with 607 in the primary care group. The researchers concluded that, "The exercise class was more clinically effective than traditional practitioner management . . . and was cost effective."

INCREASE YOUR MENTAL ACUITY. Women may experience memory loss or disturbed concentration during menopause. Sometimes this happens because of hormonal imbalance, poor health, depression, or medications. But unless there's irreversible brain damage, physical activity can invigorate and revitalize the mind. Aerobic exercise helps move blood and oxygen to all the body's organs, including the brain.

One study followed 132 people between the ages of 24 and 76. All the participants were tested for intelligence, verbal memory, and simple and complex cognitive speed. Researchers found improvements in mental sharpness after these individuals increased their aerobic activity.

LOSE WEIGHT. One obvious benefit of exercise is weight loss. You have got to move to burn up those calories. More than that, exercise stimulates your body's metabolic centers to turn on the "fat burners." Many of my perimenopausal and menopausal patients feel that body weight suddenly began to pile on after the onset of the "change of life." Yet when they analyze how much they actually exercise each day, it becomes evident that they can't blame what's happening entirely on dietary imbalances and hormone changes.

Of course, exercise will invariably build or tone muscle, which not only increases your strength, but boosts your metabolism as well. Even when resting, an efficient metabolism converts more calories to energy.

Other Exercise Perks

The habit of consistent physical activity can be a healthful substitute for negative habits. In fact, when people start exercising regularly, they often quit smoking, reduce their alcohol consumption, and become more conscientious about nutrition and weight control. An exercise program can trigger a cascade of healthy choices.

Here are a few other ways in which exercise can improve your day-to-day life:

1. **Sociability.** Many people enjoy going to exercise classes and gyms because of the social contact. Working out together promotes camaraderie. In addition, friends who exercise together can also share encouragement, direction, and support.

2. **Recreation.** When you choose a workout you enjoy, you're treating yourself by taking time out of a busy day to do something fun.

3. **Diversion.** Exercise is a "time out" with positive results. As author Joan Borysenko points out, "There is a direct correlation between how tense the muscles are and how fast the mind runs. When you pay attention to the feeling in your muscles, you're not looking so hard at the garbage in your mind."

4. **Quality of life.** Exercise works to increase strength, flexibility, endurance, coordination, agility, speed, timing, and balance. All of these work to improve the quality of one's life.

CUSTOMIZING YOUR EXERCISE PROGRAM

It is important to individualize the duration and intensity of your workouts, based on your overall health and how fit you currently are. Also, your menotype classification often helps dictate what your exercise program should be.

For example, menotype A's, if in shape, can exercise at will and usually feel much better from it. Menotype B's, if in shape, do well with exercise but some women in this category need to start slowly, due to perimenopause-associated symptoms such as bleeding fibroids, cramping, and so on. Menotype C's really require exercise due to their increased probability of osteoporosis. However, if a perimenopausal C is experiencing heavy, uterine bleeding, then intense and long bouts of exercise is not recommended.

FINDING THE RIGHT EXERCISE

People often have a preconceived notion of what exercise really is. Most of us have been programmed to think that exercise is some type of orga-

THE PREFERENCE GAME

Pay attention to which activities you like and which you don't. If you hate swimming, then joining a pool is not going to get you to swim, even though it's great exercise. If you love to walk, then walk! Whatever you do is up to you, so long as you do it consistently and with enough intensity to make it a challenge.

How do you know when you've finally found the right activities? Ask yourself the following questions:

1. Do I enjoy this exercise and feel comfortable with it?

2. Do I feel better for an extended period after the workout, like the rest of the day or even longer?

3. Do I feel benefits at low doses, that is, does my mood lift even when I work out for short periods?

When you can answer YES to these questions, you've got the exercise that's perfect for you.

nized sport, such as basketball, racquetball, or running, or something that must make you feel pain to realize any health benefit.

Clear your mind of these thoughts and replace them with this one: "Exercise is simply my body in motion."

Choose activities that you enjoy. You're not so likely to stick with something that isn't fun. Remember, exercise can take many forms: walking, lifting weights, swimming or water exercises, riding a stationary bicycle, dancing, cross-country skiing, using a rowing machine, and aerobics classes to name just a few.

Make your own list of enjoyable activities that put your body in motion. For example, we have some patients who dance for one to two hours two to three times a week. The trick is that they dance without taking a break. As long as you're not standing around talking most of the time, you are exercising.

A MOVER'S BEST FRIEND

It could be listening to music. It could be the company of a friend. It could be getting to the tea shop on the other side of town. Find a way to combine things you enjoy with your exercise activity and you'll achieve your goal with no hardship. So pick up your Walkman, stop by a friend's house to invite her along, then take a brisk walk, and treat yourselves to a cup of tea!

List the top five here and review them each month to make sure you are on the right track.

1. _____

2. _____

3. _____

4. _____

5. _____

Be sure to consider your goals when choosing your activity. What results do you want from your exercise? Your answer might include things like weight loss, increased energy, stress reduction, more time spent outdoors, and so on.

THE EXERCISE YOU HARDLY NOTICE

You can get plenty of exercise during your normal, daily schedule. Taking the stairs instead of the elevator, walking instead of driving, raking leaves, playing with young children, and gardening all contribute to great fitness. There are even studies that show cleaning the house can yield significant fitness benefits if you work hard while you're doing it.

EXERCISE EVALUATION

Circle YES or NO for each of the following ten statements. Then read the evaluation of your exercise routine.

1.	I am not exercising at all.	YES	NO
2.	I exercise less than three times a week.	YES	NO
3.	I exercise at least three times a week.	YES	NO
4.	I feel great after I workout.	YES	NO
5.	I am meeting my exercise goals.	YES	NO
6.	I enjoy working out.	YES	NO
7.	I feel tired all the time.	YES	NO
8.	My muscles and joints are constantly sore.	YES	NO
9.	My exercise routine has become boring.	YES	NO
10.	My endurance and/or strength is not improving.	YES	NO

Evaluation:

❦ If you answered YES to either #1 or #2, you need to exercise more. Go to the following "Just Getting Started" section.

ᴥ If you answered YES to #3, #4, #5, and #6, you are likely doing a beneficial exercise routine. Go to the "Maintainers" section.

ᴥ If you answered YES to #7, #8, #9, or #10, go to the "Temporary Decreasers" section. Please note that answering YES to #7 (feeling tired all the time) can also be related to not exercising enough, so also read the "Just Getting Started" section.

ᴥ If you answered NO to #3, go to the "Just Getting Started" section.

ᴥ If you answered NO to #4, go to the "Temporary Decreasers" section as well as the previous section entitled "Finding the Right Exercise."

ᴥ If you answered NO to #5, you either need to reevaluate your goals to make sure they are realistic or review the "Temporary Decreasers" section.

ᴥ If you answered NO to #6, go to the "Temporary Decreasers" section as well as the previous section entitled "Finding the Right Exercise."

Just Getting Started

The following program is for people who are thinking about starting or have just started an exercise program. It takes at least two weeks to get used to any new exercise program, so it's a good idea to ask for the encouragement and support of a close friend or relative during this time.

If you are a menotype B or C and coping with some significant adjustments due to your menopausal transition, you will probably not want to go beyond this level of exercise.

1. Choose an activity that you enjoy, such as walking, swimming, aerobics, tennis, bike riding, and so on.

2. Purchase a quality pair of shoes (proper fit and shock absorbency) and clothing for the particular exercise you are going to get involved with.

3. Choose a time of day you are most likely to exercise.

4. Limber up for 5 minutes before starting your exercise. For example, before you go walking, lift your knees up to your waist a few times, rotate your ankles, and do some light stretches.

5. Exercise for 15 minutes a day, 3 days a week for the first 2 weeks.

6. After the initial 2 weeks, gradually (over the next 4 weeks) increase the amount of time you exercise to 30 minutes. Within three months of beginning your exercise program, you should try to exercise for 30 to 60 minutes per session. In addition, the frequency should be a minimum of three days but try for five.

NOTE: Be sure to drink filtered water before and after your exercise. Also, try and wait at least one hour after eating before exercising and eat a snack or meal within an hour after exercising to maintain blood-sugar levels (should include a protein and complex carbohydrate source).

Maintainers

If you found yourself in this category, that is a good sign. It means you are probably on a consistent program that consists of 30 to 60 minutes of activity done 3 to 5 times a week. You feel good, and you're meeting your fitness goals.

The biggest risk for women in this group is that you can become bored or lose motivation to continue with your program over time. To help prevent this, I recommend reading and incorporating some of the suggestions in the later section entitled "Staying Motivated."

Temporary Decreasers

If you found yourself answering YES to #7, #8, #9, and #10 in the exercise evaluation, you may be overtraining. This means your body is not recovering fully from the exercise you are doing. The tissues in your muscles are not healing, and you may be "taxing" your ability to produce stress hormones such as cortisol and DHEA. A health trainer or physician can help ascertain whether overtraining is a problem for you.

What causes overtraining? Your exercise routine may be too long (for example, 2 hours) or too frequent (7 days a week), or you may be exercising when it's inappropriate, such as when you have a cold or bronchitis.

Signs and symptoms of too much exercise can include but are not limited to:

Depression

Frequent injuries

Low libido

Weight loss (beyond normal weight loss)

Insomnia

If you're in this category, you need to decrease the duration and/or frequency of workouts by 50 percent for 3 to 4 weeks. During that time, you may find that your energy levels increase and the chronic muscle soreness goes away. After 4 weeks you can increase your exercise level (duration and frequency) by 25 percent, but do not go back to the level that caused the problem in the first place.

STAYING MOTIVATED

Plenty of people start exercising, but few stick with it. Research has shown that about half of those who begin an exercise program drop out within 6 to 12 months.

Here are some tips for staying motivated:

- **Envision success.** In your mind's eye, see yourself enjoying exercise and the remarkable benefits that it brings.

- **Do it for yourself.** The best motivation comes from within. It's okay to seek motivation from family, friends, and other resources, but your biggest motivation should be to please yourself.

- **Do it together.** Working out with others doubles the chance that you will stick with it. It also makes exercise more fun.

- **Pat yourself on the back.** Set goals, and reward yourself when you've accomplished them. For example, if you lose ten pounds, treat yourself to a professional massage.

- **Tell everybody about your plans.** Share your goals with friends and families. Put your plan in writing: what exercises you'll be doing and how often you'll do them. It may take six months for exercise to become an ingrained, permanent habit.

- **Be realistic.** Instead of striving to look like a supermodel, focus on greater strength and increased stamina. If weight loss is your primary motivation, try to lose one pound a week if you have a lot of weight to lose.

- **Change the time you exercise.** If you can't roll out of bed for a 6 A.M. exercise class, a lunch-time walk may be more realistic. Perhaps working out at the end of the day is best for you.

- **Keep a journal.** Keep a log of the days you exercised, what you did, and how you felt. This will help to keep you on track and focused.

- **Try something new.** If you're bored with your usual workout, then it's time to broaden your options. Have you tried free weights? Rowing machines? Dancing? Swimming? An enjoyable new activity can spark your interest in exercise again.

- **Use the power of music.** Music can be powerfully motivating while exercising. It helps take your mind off physical exertion and provides more pleasure. I love to listen to my favorite tunes while on a "power walk" or jogging.

- **Use pictures.** If you have lost weight since beginning your exercise program, for example, then put a picture of your "old" and "new" self in a place where you will see it often, such as a mirror.

- **Pray about it.** Seek higher guidance to strengthen your commitment and motivation.

SHE TRIED IT

Dianne, 48, was beginning to feel a sensation of sadness during menopause. I talked with her about her feelings, as well as her lifestyle, then recommended she start walking each morning before work. To keep her motivated, I suggested she take a Walkman and listen to her favorite music, which for her happened to be Faith Hill. She started the next morning. Later, she admitted that staying consistent for the first two weeks was tough, but she stuck with her program. Dianne walked for 30 minutes five mornings a week. Before long, she noticed her spirits starting to lift. Soon, her sadness and depression had gone away. She even lost a little bit of weight, which was a bonus. Dianne feels so motivated by her progress that she now swims in addition to her daily walks.

EVALUATING ACHES AND PAINS

Once you've started a program, you will invariably feel some muscle soreness and tightness, especially for the first two weeks. This is normal. With rest, stretching, proper nutrition, and recuperative techniques like massage and saunas, your soreness, tightness, and aches should dissipate.

After about two weeks, you'll notice the soreness going away more quickly after exercise, generally within two to three days. After another month or so, recovery time will drop to one or two days. If it doesn't, it is a sign that you are:

1. **Overtraining.** You're exercising for too long a time or too intensely.

2. **Nutritionally deficient.** Your diet may be lacking in quality protein, complex carbohydrates, certain vitamins and minerals, or essential fatty acids, thereby preventing tissue repair.

3. **Exercising or stretching incorrectly.** Consult with a fitness trainer for coaching.

4. **Requiring some extra recuperation.** Inadequate sleep can prevent your body from recovering. If you do sleep well at night, consider a 30-minute "siesta" during the day. Also, you may need to try restorative techniques such as massage, chiropractic, acupuncture, or saunas. If you are exercising six to seven days a week, you may need to take an extra day off once in awhile to allow more time for tissue repair.

WHEN YOU NEED MEDICAL HELP

See your doctor if you experience the following:

- Muscle or joint pain that is extreme or restricts motion and/or does not improve within five days.

- Injuries sustained while exercising. For example, sprained ankle, neck or back injury, or others that do not seem to be part of the normal wear and tear of exercise.

- Shortness of breath, dizziness, or chest pain before, during, or after exercise.

EXERCISE BEYOND MENOPAUSE

Both the World Health Organization and the National Institutes of Health recommend that clinicians encourage all patients to enroll in an exercise program. Consistent physical activity reduces the risk of heart disease and premature death.

One study focused on 40,417 postmenopausal Iowa women, average age 69. A mailed questionnaire assessed their physical activity. Researchers found that, in general, the more frequent and intense the activity, the lower the risk of mortality. These findings support the claim that postmenopausal women who engage in regular physical activity may reduce their mortality risk.

BENEFITS OF STRENGTH TRAINING

Once thought of as strictly a form of exercise for males, strength-training techniques, such as weight lifting, have begun to enjoy popularity among women, and for good reason.

As you age, you lose muscle fibers, and the ones you retain become smaller, as well as less receptive to messages from your central nervous system. The combination of these factors impairs strength, balance, and coordination. In addition, as you lose muscle mass, you are likely to gain body fat.

However, no matter how old you are, strength training can help slow down—and possibly reverse—your loss of muscle mass and strength. That's one reason the American College of Sports Medicine's fitness guidelines now recommend strength training for people over 50, along with aerobic exercise and stretching.

One review looked at several studies on strength training among older people. The authors of the review concluded that strength training increases the strength, mass, power, and quality of skeletal muscle. In addition, it can increase endurance, lower blood pressure in individuals with hypertension, and reduce insulin resistance. Strength training also decreases body fat, protects against the loss of bone mineral density, reduces the risk of falling, may alleviate pain and improve function in osteoarthritic knee joints, and can help you to recover more quickly from injuries.

With stronger muscles, you can carry groceries, move furniture, put items on high shelves, and lift small children with greater ease and less pain.

Consider a University of Alabama at Birmingham study on older women and weight lifting. Fourteen healthy women, 60 to 77 years old, lifted weights for one hour, three times a week, for 16 weeks. At the end of the study, the women were able to carry bags of groceries with 36-percent less effort, and to get up from their chairs with 40-percent less stress on their leg muscles.

Before You Start Lifting Weights

Because of the risk for injury, approach weight training with respect. Personal trainers are available at many gyms and health clubs to help you get started. Or, if you know someone with an expertise in resistance training, ask for help. Also consider the following:

- **Use machines.** If you're a beginner, exercise machines may be your best choice. These machines use weights and pulleys to provide resistance. They're easier and safer to use than free weights. The only drawback is that you usually have to belong to a gym or health club to use exercise machines, unless you can afford to buy your own—and the good ones are expensive.

- **Warm up before you lift weights.** If you exercise aerobically and lift weights on the same day, do your aerobics first. That will help warm up your body and decrease your risk of injury.

- **Don't work the same muscles two days in a row.** Rest for one full day between exercising each specific muscle group. Some people do a complete session of weight training every other day. Others work on upper body muscles one day and lower body muscles the next.

- **Go from big to little.** Work on the large muscle groups—such as the quadriceps—first, and save the small muscle groups—such as the forearms—for last. The large muscle groups help get the blood circulating.

- **Breathe properly.** While working against resistance, breathe out on the hard part, and breathe in on the easy part. When you hold your breath for long periods of time, you're withholding oxygen from the brain.

- **Don't rush.** Perform strength exercises slowly and precisely. Quality counts more than quantity.

- **Check with your doctor.** Do not start strength training without your healthcare practitioner's consent if you have high blood pressure. Strength training, especially isometric contractions, can temporarily raise blood pressure.

• **Stop when it hurts.** Do not continue any exercise that causes pain or discomfort.

THE APPEAL OF WALKING

Walking is the easiest, safest, most effective, and most affordable form of exercise. Anyone, at any age, with a working pair of legs and good shoes can walk for fitness. You don't need to join a health club, get special training, or buy expensive equipment. Regular, brisk walks boost cardiovascular health, raise the percentage of lean body mass (while burning up fat), and help keep bones strong. Walk at a brisk pace so that you're breathing a little harder, but never so hard that you can't hold a conversation. As with any exercise, if you start to feel dizzy, sick, or experience any unusual pain, stop what you're doing and get to a health-care professional.

BALANCE YOUR PROGRAM

A well-rounded exercise program includes strength/resistance training, stretching, and aerobics.

If you decide to start working out with weights, first learn the correct technique from a professional. If you don't lift the right way, you can injure yourself.

Stretching before a workout reduces your risk of injury and muscle strain. Stretching improves flexibility, increases blood flow, and gets the body ready for exercise. It should be an integral part of warming up and cooling down.

As for aerobic exercise, people over 50 may be more comfortable with some form of non-jarring activity, such as walking, swimming, cycling, or low-impact dancing.

PROCEED WITH CAUTION

It is always advisable to consult with your physician before embarking on an exercise program. It's particularly important to check with your doctor if you're seriously overweight, habitually sedentary, a smoker, or are planning to work with weights for the first time.

In addition, always check with your doctor if you have high blood pressure; heart trouble; diabetes; a family history of strokes or heart attacks; frequent dizzy spells; extreme breathlessness upon minor exertion; arthritis or other bone problems; severe muscular, ligament, or tendon problems; or any known or suspected diseases or conditions, including back problems.

If you've already started an exercise program, there may be times when you need to stop and consult a healthcare professional. For example, if you develop sudden pain, shortness of breath, or feel ill, stop exercising immediately and see your doctor. The same is true if you experience pressure or discomfort in your chest, faintness, rapid or irregular heartbeat, excessive fatigue, or severe joint or muscle pain.

WHERE TO FIND SUITABLE EXERCISE PROGRAMS

To find an exercise program that suits your interests and abilities, contact your local health club, university, or hospital. In addition, YMCAs, YWCAs, senior and civic centers, parks, recreation programs, churches and synagogues, and shopping malls often organize exercise, wellness, or walking programs.

Almost every individual can find some way to become more active. Find what works for you, and discover how much younger and stronger you feel in a matter of weeks. You can single-handedly minimize menopausal symptoms, strengthen your bones and heart, naturally relieve pain, improve your quality of sleep, sharpen your mind, lift your mood, and reduce your risk of diabetes. You may live longer, and you'll definitely live better.

20 RANDOM ACTS OF EXERCISE

Following are 20 creative tips to help you get regular exercise.

1. **Use creative TV watching.** When watching television, ride a stationary bike or walk on the spot. Time goes by very quickly this way and it prevents you from becoming a "couch potato."

2. **Choose stairs instead of an elevator.** This really burns up the calories and works the heart. You don't have to go fast. A smooth pace will get the blood moving.

3. **Move your arms as you walk.** Pretend you are swimming or lifting weights. Sounds strange but you get twice the workout by involving both the legs and upper body.

4. **Take fitness breaks.** If you use the computer a lot at work or home, take a break every hour and do five to ten minutes of exercise. It will also help prevent neck and back problems.

5. **Walk a pet or a baby stroller.** If you do not have a dog or baby, ask to join a neighbor on a stroll with his or her dog or baby. Or borrow a pet to walk if you don't have one of your own.

6. **Bike it.** If it is not too far, ride your bike to work or to a friend's home on a regular basis.

7. **Make your VCR an exercise machine.** Instead of a regular movie, rent an exercise video. This will get you physically involved with the "action."

8. **Use the "power of two."** Schedule morning or after-work walks with a friend. You can have a nice conversation while getting some exercise.

9. **Wash your car instead of using the carwash.** It is a good body workout and will save you money!

10. **Make your garden grow.** If you are not already doing so, get involved with regular gardening at your home. It is more physically challenging than you think—plus you get to enjoy the outdoors.

11. **Knock down some pins.** Go bowling with your family or friends. It's fun and involves some physical activity.

12. **Join a women's aqua-aerobics class.** This is a great way to get exercise that is easy on the joints. Plus, you'll meet some new friends.

13. **Go mall walking.** You get to enjoy looking at all the window specials while getting exercise.

14. **Stretch at every opportunity.** Stretch while the copier is running or while the coffee is brewing. Stretching helps to reduce pain, reduces risk of injury, prevents muscle spasms and cramps, and improves blood flow.

15. **Do some morning crunches.** Start with two sets of ten crunches when you get up each morning. Increase the number over time. You'll feel good for the rest of the day, knowing that you're toning up those abs.

16. **Mow the lawn.** Give your husband or kids a shock and tell them you are going to mow the lawn. While not glamorous, it can be a good workout.

17. **Put on weight.** Wear ankle weights as you do housework.

18. **Ditch the wheels.** Park in the farthest parking spot when you go shopping.

19. **Go outside and play.** Take a walk or play catch or kickball with your kids or grandkids.

20. **Be a helper.** Volunteer at a nursing care center to push wheelchair-bound people outdoors.

9

$\mathcal{P}$UTTING IT ALL TOGETHER

$\mathcal{E}$ven after you begin to experience success in dealing with your symptoms and to feel more comfortable, you'll still need to monitor and rebalance yourself once in awhile. But this isn't so difficult as it sounds. I'll guide you through an overall "plan," but with what you've read in the preceding chapters, you already have the knowledge you need to make adjustments. Of course, you'll continue to see the doctor or practitioner you've selected, who will help you. And remember, it's a good idea to keep a journal, which can alert you to areas of your health or lifestyle that need attention.

Here are three-month recommendations for each menotype. *All* menotypes should read the menotype-A program. Menotypes B and C should read the B program. Only Menotype C's need to read the C program.

MENOTYPE-A PROGRAM

Month 1

Nutrition

ช *Pay attention to the amount of plant foods in your diet.* Naturally occurring phytosterols and phytoestrogens found in soy and many vegetables have a balancing effect on your hormones and may also prevent hormone-dependent tumors such as breast cancer. You should be shooting for seven servings of fruits and vegetables daily. Start by having a large salad or serving of steamed vegetables with lunch and dinner.

*   *Cut down on sugars and refined carbohydrates.* This includes such obvious foods as table sugar, soda, candy bars, and less obvious foods such as crackers, white bread, and non-whole grain pastas. Reducing the amount of sugar in your diet will help prevent heart disease and possibly cancer, improve your energy level, balance your moods, and make it easier for you to lose weight or prevent weight gain.

*   *Cut down on red meat and dairy products and increase your intake of fermented soy products.* Try adding tofu, miso, and other soy products to your meals. Unless you are vegetarian, consume fish (salmon, mackerel, and so on) two to three times weekly. Focus on consuming a quality protein source, such as legumes, nuts, seeds, soy, fish, and lean poultry, with your meals and snacks.

*   *Use extra virgin olive oil instead of other cooking oils.* Olive oil is much healthier for your heart. It is excellent to use in your salad dressing as well.

*   *Increase your water intake.* Drink at least 48 ounces of water daily (six 8-ounce glasses). If you drink more than two cups of coffee a day, then start replacing the extra cups with green tea or other herbal teas (chamomile, peppermint, and so on).

*   *Go organic.* Make a conscious decision to use organic foods as much as possible. It is not only better for your body, but good for the planet as well.

Exercise

*   *Begin your exercise program with an activity you enjoy.* Think deeply about this because the exercise you choose will greatly influence whether you continue exercising over the long term or not. (Of course, a positive attitude and high motivation toward exercise are most important.)

> ❧ *Find an exercise partner.* This could be a friend or a pet who can make walking and some other exercise more enjoyable.

> ❧ *See your doctor.* If you have not had much physical activity in awhile, it's always a good idea to have a check-up with your doctor first before starting any exercise program.

> ❧ *Begin slowly.* Start at 15 minutes three times a week. For those who desire a trainer, I say go for it. The right person will help you stay motivated and design a program specific for you.

Supplements

> ❧ *Take a multi.* Start on a high-potency multivitamin without iron (unless your doctor has determined your blood levels of iron are low).

> ❧ *Use calcium.* Unless your multivitamin contains 1,000 mg in a good form, you should be taking calcium in a supplemental dosage of 500 mg daily. Look for the calcium citrate or citrate-malate form that also contains additional magnesium (for a daily total close to 250 mg).

> ❧ *Add vitamin E.* If your multivitamin does not contain 400 IU of vitamin E, then consider taking a separate supplement.

> ❧ *Take EFA's.* Essential fatty acids may be needed if you do not consume much cold-water fish or nuts. I recommend either a high-quality fish oil (3,000 mg) or one tablespoon of flaxseed oil. You can also use an essential fatty acid blend that contains a mixture of the different essential fatty acids.

> ❧ *Use Black Cohosh.* If you are having mild or infrequent menopausal symptoms and want to take something, then I recommend using a herb such as Black Cohosh. Start at 80 mg daily of a 2.5% triterpene glycoside standardized extract. It can be taken by itself or with other menopausal herbs as listed in Chapter 3.

❧ *Try homeopathy.* Another good option is to use homeopathy, which can relieve symptoms and prevent them from causing problems in the future.

Lifestyle

❧ *See an acupuncturist.* Acupuncture from a qualified practitioner can be helpful in relieving symptoms.

❧ *Relax.* Take 15 minutes a day for relaxation or meditation. You can try techniques such as mental imagery (envisioning positive pictures in your mind), prayer, and so on.

Month 2

Nutrition

❧ *Continue to increase the amounts of vegetables, fruits, nuts, seeds, whole grains, and legumes in your diet.* Now is also a great time to add flaxseeds to your diet. This is an incredibly powerful way to increase fiber in your diet, and consume cardiovascular and immune-system protective omega-3 fatty acids and phytonutrients.

❧ *Increase your supplemental calcium.* Bring it to a total (multivitamin and/or separate calcium supplement total combined) of 1,000 mg daily and your magnesium dose to 500 mg.

Supplements

❧ *Continue your program.* If you are using Black Cohosh or some of the other menopausal herbs, you should be noticing some improvements by now. Continue on the same dosage as recommended for month 1.

❧ *Try memory supplements.* If your memory is not so good as you would like it to be, then consider using Ginkgo biloba (180 to 240 mg daily of a 24% extract) or the brain nutrient Phosphatidylserine (200 to 300 mg daily).

≈ *Consider heart supplements.* If cholesterol and other cardio-vascular risk markers are a factor, then use the supplements specific for you. For example, if you have elevated homocysteine levels, then extra B vitamins as described in Chapter 10 are recommended. High cholesterol levels can usually be managed with exercise, diet, and supplements such as niacin, guggulipid, and antioxidants.

Exercise

≈ *Add time.* If you are feeling comfortable with your exercise progress, then increase your time to 30 to 45 minutes per session. This will help continue your progress and fitness level.

Lifestyle

≈ *Relax even more.* Increase your relaxation time to 15 to 30 minutes daily. Your health, peace of mind, and soul are worth it.

Month 3

Nutrition

≈ *Try new foods.* Experiment with variety in your diet. Try new recipes (healthy ones) so that you get a fuller array of nutrients in your body. Variety will also help to prevent problems with food sensitivities. Now is a good time to look through your refrigerator, cupboards, and food pantry. They should be stocked with fewer packaged, processed foods and more fresh, unprocessed foods. The word "organic" should appear often, especially on fruits and vegetables.

Supplements

≈ *Add greens.* The only addition you may want to consider supplement-wise is a source of one of the supergreen foods such as chlorella, spirulina, wheatgrass, or a blend of them and others that are commonly available. Be sure to purchase an organic product from a reputable brand.

Exercise

• *Add weights.* If not already doing so, consider adding some light weight-training to your program twice a week. You can either do this after your regular exercise routine (for example, walking) or in place of a session or two of aerobic exercise. If you have no experience with weights, consult with a trainer or friend who can make sure you are lifting the weights with proper form.

• *Take aerobics to the max.* Your aerobic exercise by this time should be approximately 45 to 60 minutes four to five times weekly.

Lifestyle

• *Relax all you can.* Put aside 30 to 60 minutes daily of quality relaxation time.

• *Check with an expert.* If you feel that your mood and energy are somewhat off and have not responded to natural therapies, consider consulting with a naturopathic doctor, holistic medical doctor, homeopath, or acupuncturist.

SHE TRIED IT

Leanna, a 50-year-old lawyer, was looking for natural options to conventional hormone replacement. Although she was having no problems with menopause, her doctor urged her to begin hormone replacement immediately to "prevent heart attacks and broken bones." After taking a thorough history, then reviewing her bone-density study, bloodwork, and saliva hormone profile, it became evident that Leanna was in the menotype-A category. I recommended that she continue her current diet and exercise program. I also recommended she start on a multivitamin, calcium/magnesium, and an antioxidant formula that included vitamin E. She continues to do well on this program.

COMMON MENOTYPE-A
QUESTIONS AND ANSWERS

Q: *I am 50 years old and have been in menopause for three months. So far I do not have any strong menopausal symptoms—hot flashes, etc., are quite bearable. My doctor told me that my bone density is quite good for my age and that I have low cardiovascular risk. However, he states that I should still take estrogen to protect my bones and heart, as it is good preventive medicine. Is that necessary?*

A: If you are a menotype A, by definition you do not require hormones. Diet, lifestyle, supplements, and stress reduction should be your focus. Hormones (especially synthetic hormones) have their own set of inherent health risks (breast cancer, and so on). In my opinion, you have a much greater probability of developing health problems if you use hormones than if you stick with the non-hormonal menotype-A program.

Q: *Recently my cycle has become irregular and I notice the occasional hot flash. Based on my assessment, I am a menotype A. I am wondering what I should take to stop the irregular cycles.*

A: Your goal should not be to stop the irregular cycles, as this is a normal part of the perimenopausal transition. However, you can use herbs (particularly Vitex) or homeopathy and supplements to prevent extremely heavy bleeding, etc.

Q: *Is it possible that I could start perimenopause / menopause as a menotype A and then later require the program for a menotype B or C?*

A: Yes, that is possible. An example might be a woman who has relatively few symptoms her first few months of menopause and then all of a sudden her symptoms (hot flashes, vaginal dryness, and so on) become overwhelming and unresponsive to the menotype-A program. In this case, a change to a menotype-B or -C program would be indicated. A menotype-A woman who, for some reason, has her ovaries removed would also find herself in the menotype-C category.

The only time I have seen a woman go from menotype C to menotype B, or menotype B or C to menotype A is when the wrong therapy was prescribed from the start. For example, one woman who came to me had no major menopausal symptoms, but her family doctor prescribed hormone replacement. Her doctor wanted to treat her as a menotype C, when she really required an A or B menotype program.

SHE TRIED IT

At the age of 49, Marcy began herbal therapy to relieve the hot flashes and night sweats that began during perimenopause. She had been doing well on the herbs for almost a year when she began to experience very strong hot flashes. An increase in the herbal dosage of Black Cohosh and other herbs was not helpful. Homeopathy and other nutritional supplements were not helpful either. A saliva hormone test showed very low estrogen levels, slightly low progesterone, and normal testosterone, DHEA, and cortisol. Due to her severe symptoms and low estrogen levels, Marcy was put on the menotype-C protocol and experienced quick improvement of her hot flashes on natural estrogen and progesterone.

MENOTYPE-B PROGRAM

Month 1

General

❧ *Follow the A plan.* Follow the same regimen (diet, exercise, herbs/supplements, and relaxation) as for menotype A for the first four weeks. The following situations need to be addressed more commonly by Menotype B's.

Supplements

❧ *Try St. John's Wort.* Depression and anxiety can be helped in most cases with herbs such as St. John's Wort (600 to 900 mg daily of a standardized product containing 0.3% hypericin and 3–5% hyperforin) or the supplement SAMe at a dosage of 400 to 800 mg.

❧ **Black Cohosh.** Take 40 mg (2.5% triterpene glycosides) twice daily to reduce hot flashes and other menopausal symptoms.

❧ **Add homeopathic remedies.** Homeopathy can be extremely helpful for these common conditions. I also find it works very well for feelings of anger and grief. Remedies such as Sepia and Ignatia can help a lot of women.

Month 2

If you have not had adequate relief of symptoms after four weeks, then make the following changes.

Supplements

❧ **Change your Black Cohosh dosage.** Increase it to 160 mg daily by taking 80 mg in the morning and 80 mg before bedtime. Some women also find this regimen helpful in relieving night sweats.

❧ **Add soy.** You should also consider taking a fermented soy protein powder, especially if you do not consume soy foods on a regular basis.

Hormone replacement

❧ **Start natural progesterone replacement therapy.** For women who still have severe symptoms involving vaginal dryness, hot flashes, insomnia, and mood problems (anxiety, depression) after four to six weeks of a non-hormone approach, the use of natural progesterone is warranted. (See Chapter 4 for dosage information.) Of course, your hormone tests will corroborate low levels of progesterone.

❧ **Check other hormone levels.** Low levels of DHEA and/or pregnenolone may be contributing to your symptoms. If testing shows low levels, supplementation under the guidance of a knowledgeable doctor can be helpful.

~~~~~~

SHE TRIED IT

Sarah, a menotype B, described her hot flashes as bothersome, especially when night came and they disrupted her sleep. A dose of 80 mg of Black Cohosh had been working well to keep the hot flashes at bay during the day, so I recommended she take an additional 80 mg before bedtime. Within two weeks, most of her nighttime hot flashes and night sweats had cleared up.

Month 3

Hormones

❧ *Go to the next level.* If you are still having night sweats, hot flashes, vaginal dryness, and other menopausal symptoms— and you are on an adequate dosage of natural progesterone or DHEA/pregnenolone—take a look at the recommendations for menotype C.

Supplements

❧ *Supplement for bone loss.* If your doctor has discovered that you have the very beginnings of bone loss (osteopenia), I recommend you also supplement with a bone formula that contains 600 mg of Ipriflavone daily. Before you start, however, have your doctor test your white blood cell count because in some cases it may cause a drop in these immune cells. Levels of the white blood cells (lymphocytes) should then be checked periodically to make sure your levels remain normal. Also, remember to take bone-building vitamins and minerals such as D, boron, silicon, and others as described in Chapter 11.

COMMON MENOPTYPE-B
QUESTIONS AND ANSWERS

Q: *I am a menotype B. Can I start on natural progesterone right away without trying herbs first?*

A: Yes, although I typically recommend herbs like Black Cohosh and Vitex first, as they are inherently safer. (They balance hormones already present in the body.) However, natural progesterone appears quite safe, especially when compared to synthetic hormones such as Premarin® and Provera®.

Q: *I have a moderate amount of vaginal dryness. Will natural progesterone be effective without my taking any estrogen?*

A: It depends on the woman. For some, it does work well; and for others, hormones such as DHEA, testosterone, or estrogen are required. It is worth trying natural progesterone by itself first. A certain amount of progesterone is converted by the body into estrogen.

Q: *Can I take Black Cohosh and other menopausal herbs in combination with natural progesterone?*

A: Yes, you can, but I don't find it necessary in most cases. Generally I use one or the other with patients, but some women do better by taking both simultaneously.

Q: *My libido seems to be in decline. Is DHEA effective for increasing libido?*

A: Yes, DHEA can be effective for many women. A certain amount is converted into testosterone, which is known to play an important role in libido. For some women, herbs like Chinese Ginseng or Damiana can also be effective.

Q: *I am perimenopausal and experiencing heavy flow. My doctor recently told me I am anemic. What do you recommend?*

A: Assuming your doctor has ruled out other causes of vaginal bleeding, I recommend you start on either the herb Vitex or natural progesterone cream (one-quarter [20 mg] teaspoon twice daily, but stop during the flow). Depending on your cycle, your doctor can help guide you on progesterone dosage. I would also recommend taking iron in the chelated form such as citrate or glycinate (50 to 100 mg daily depending on the severity of the anemia). Vitamin C also enhances absorption when taken at the same time (250 mg), as does the herb Yellow Dock (two capsules or 30 drops twice daily) and the homeopathic Ferrum Phos 3X or 6X (five pellets three times daily). Iron-deficiency anemia can in itself lead to heavier bleeding.

Q: *I have a history of drinking and smoking. Will this affect my menopausal transition, and, if so, what can I do about it?*

A: Smoking, excess alcohol, drugs, stress, and environmental pollution all tax the liver. The liver metabolizes all the hormones in the body, so if it is not working optimally, it can lead to hormone-imbalance problems. Herbs such as Milk Thistle, Globe Artichoke, Dandelion Root, and Burdock Root are excellent in helping cleanse the liver and restoring its function. They can be taken individually or as part of herbal liver formulas. Vitamin C, magnesium, lipoic acid, vitamin E, green tea, and several other common supplements also help to improve liver function.

MENOTYPE-C PROGRAM

Month 1

Nutrition

• *Follow the A–B plan.* Dietary recommendations are the same as for menotypes A and B. Review them above.

ﻬ *Get the bone destroyers off your plate.* If you have osteoporosis, it is imperative that you focus on cutting out or greatly reducing foods that lead to bone loss such as caffeine, alcohol, salt, sugar, and red meat.

ﻬ *Increase foods that build strong bones.* To review, these include omega-3-rich fish such as salmon, mackerel, and herring, as well as bone-healthy foods such as soy, broccoli, kale, and the many sea vegetables.

Exercise

ﻬ *Start your exercise program the same as for menotypes A and B.* However, if you have moderate to severe osteoporosis, then it is important to incorporate weight-bearing exercise—such as walking and the use of weights—into your program. If you are just starting your exercise program, the use of weights should be slowly introduced over time with the help of a trainer.

Supplements

ﻬ *Add phytonutrients.* Indole-3 carbinole and d-glucarate are two of the better ones to help with hormone detoxification. (By definition, menotype C women are on hormone replacement.) I recommend women use supplements like these to help prevent the build-up of toxic hormone metabolites that may cause hormone-dependent tumors such as breast cancer.

ﻬ *Supplement with a bone formula that contains 600 mg of Ipriflavone.* Follow the same recommendations given for menotype-B women using this supplement.

Hormones

ﻬ *Change to the naturals.* If you are one of the many women on a synthetic estrogen replacement such as Premarin®, I recommend working with a doctor who will help you make the transition to natural hormone replacement. Your hormone analysis will help decide whether hormones other than estrogen and progesterone (testosterone, DHEA, thyroid, and so on) should be used. For women who have severe osteoporosis, I recommend having their IgF-1 levels tested to get an idea of their growth-hormone levels.

Month 2

General

- ❧ *Be patient.* If you have made the switch to natural hormone replacement and do not feel "quite right" yet, do not worry. It can take a month or more for your body to adjust and your doctor to find the right dose and delivery system of natural hormones for you. Keep a diet diary and tell your doctor what you are experiencing. Your symptoms as well as lab testing will help to fine-tune your hormone prescription.

- ❧ *Retest your bones.* Have your bone-resorption test redone near the end of your second month. You want to make sure you are not breaking down bone more quickly than you are making it. Be sure you are getting proper levels of the vitamins and minerals. Absorption may also be an issue, so start taking two digestive enzymes along with a digestive herbal formula or betaine HCL with each meal.

Hormones

- ❧ *Consider taking melatonin.* If insomnia has been a problem and it has not improved with herbs (such as Passionflower, Hops, or Valerian) or other natural treatments (such as homeopathy and acupuncture), then you may require melatonin. This hormone can be measured through saliva testing. If low, then melatonin therapy can be quite effective. A good starting dose is 0.3 to 0.5 mg.

Month 3

General

- ❧ *Make an assessment.* By this time your natural hormone replacement should be working and making you feel good. Repeat testing can confirm that your hormone levels are in the normal range. This is also a good time to focus on your digestive health. If your digestion is not so strong as it should be, then probiotics, enzymes, and digestive herbs can be of benefit as described in Chapter 7. If you are not doing well, then something is wrong with either the type, dosage, and/or the delivery system of the hormones you are taking. Consult with a doctor knowledgeable in natural hormone replacement to figure out what will work better for you.

SHE TRIED IT

Valerie, a menotype C with moderate osteoporosis, came to our clinic to find out more about natural hormone replacement. She had been on Premarin® for almost two years, and although it greatly reduced her hot flashes, she thought it was making her more irritable and moody. When switched to natural estrogen, progesterone, and DHEA, she felt a tremendous improvement in her mood. She also noticed that her hair looked more full and healthy. She continues to do well on these natural alternatives.

COMMON MENOTYPE-C QUESTIONS AND ANSWERS

Q: *There are so many delivery systems of hormones—capsules, gels, creams, etc. What form of hormone replacement do you recommend I use?*

A: Women generally prefer the oil capsule form for women who need full hormone replacement and natural progesterone cream for women who only need progesterone.

Q: *I feel fine on Premarin® and want to stay on it. I have added natural progesterone to my protocol. Should I stay on the same dose of Premarin®?*

A: Since some progesterone is converted to estrogen, it is common that the dose of Premarin® be cut down, sometimes by as much as 50 percent. Work with your doctor on this adjustment. Hormone testing can be valuable in gauging your estrogen levels.

Q: *I have had breast cancer in the past yet require hormonal support because I have osteoporosis. What do you recommend?*

A: There is no definitive answer to this question. Some doctors use estriol in combination with natural progesterone. However, it is not well studied with regard to breast cancer. If hormones are used, then it is imperative for your doctor to monitor you closely.

Q: *Now that I have switched over from synthetic to natural estrogen / progesterone replacement, do you think my thyroid function will improve?*

A: Possibly. I have seen the thyroid function of many women improve when they have gotten off synthetic estrogen, which has a suppressive effect on the thyroid. You may still require thyroid hormone but in a lower amount. Testing thyroid-hormone levels as well as monitoring your body temperature will help you judge the state of your thyroid.

Q: *I have been on hormone replacement for over six months and still have problems with vaginal dryness. What do you recommend?*

A: Estriol vaginal cream from your doctor works well. At a dosage of 0.5 mg per gram of cream, insert one gram of cream daily for one to two weeks, and then reduce frequency to one or two times a week.

Q: *Once I start on hormone replacement, do I need to be on it forever?*

A: If you are on hormone replacement due to severe menopausal symptoms but have good bone density, then you can come off the hormones at some point in the future. The time depends on the woman. Some need the hormones to keep symptoms at bay for a year or two, while others need them longer. At some time in the future, you can work with your doctor to get off the hormones. If you have moderate to severe osteoporosis or some other situation that requires constant hormone replacement, you may need to be on hormones indefinitely.

10

$\mathcal{H}$EART DISEASE
AND MENOPAUSE

$\mathcal{E}$very year almost 960,000 Americans die of cardiovascular disease. It accounts for approximately 41 percent of the total deaths in the United States. Of this number 250,000 are women. Black women have twice the risk of dying from coronary artery disease as white women do.

All three menotypes are at risk. You can't count on hormone replacement therapy to protect you, and having low cholesterol doesn't necessarily mean you have nothing to worry about. Heart health is a complex issue. So what do you do?

THE HEART OF A WOMAN

Following are some women-specific statistics about heart disease from the American Heart Association.

- About 19,457 women under age 65 die of coronary heart disease each year; more than 33% of them are under age 55.
- 44% of women who have heart attacks die within a year of the event, compared to 27% of men.
- Among 63% of women who died suddenly of coronary heart disease, there was no previous evidence of disease.

CONVENTIONAL APPROACH

In a nutshell, the standard Western approach to preventing heart disease in women includes the following:

- ❧ low-fat diet rich in fruits and vegetables

- ❧ regular exercise

- ❧ abstinence from smoking

- ❧ blood testing for cholesterol levels and, in certain cases, a recommendation to use cholesterol-lowering drugs

- ❧ testing for high blood pressure and, in certain cases, a recommendation to use hypertensive medications

- ❧ estrogen replacement for menopausal and postmenopausal women

While there is scientific support for this approach, it does not address many of the factors that can cause heart disease. Many women find that nontoxic nutritional supplements and holistic approaches are just as good as or more effective than many commonly prescribed pharmaceuticals in reducing their risk.

The good news is that the Nurses' Health Study demonstrated how diet and lifestyle play major roles in the development of coronary heart disease. The authors of this study concluded, "Among women, adherence to lifestyle guidelines involving diet, exercise, and abstinence from smoking is associated with a very low risk of coronary heart disease."

RISK FACTORS

When people think about risk factors for heart disease, the first word that comes to mind is often "cholesterol." Unfortunately, cholesterol is not the only marker you need to monitor, and it may not even be the most important one. Although your cholesterol count is part of the picture, keep in mind that over half the people who die from heart disease have normal cholesterol levels.

Following is a broader picture of the risk factors you should keep in mind to maintain a healthy heart.

Total Cholesterol

Cholesterol is a yellow, waxy substance that is essential for life. It is an important component of every cell in your body. Your cells need it to function properly, and your body needs it to produce hormones. Interestingly, unoxidized cholesterol actually protects cell membranes from free-radical damage and cancer.

Although cholesterol is present in some foods we eat, approximately 80 to 85 percent of cholesterol in your body is manufactured by your liver and, to a lesser degree, the cells of your small intestine. Generally speaking, the higher the cholesterol levels, the higher the cardiovascular risk. The Framingham study found that people with cholesterol levels below 175 mg/dl had less than half the rate of heart attack as those whose levels were 250 to 275 mg/dl.

However, we must keep in mind that oxidation of cholesterol is the real issue in the development of atherosclerosis (hardening of the arteries) and heart disease. Oxidation, particularly of LDL cholesterol, initiates an inflammatory response in the blood vessel walls that causes plaque formation.

Remember, total cholesterol is just one of several markers for cardiovascular risk, and is not considered the most important marker.

Healthy value

> Below 180 (although normal is considered below 200)

Natural solutions

> Exercise.

> Flaxseed. (See the "Heart-Healthy Diet" section later in this chapter.)

> Niacin in the flush-free form of niacin known as inositol hexaniacinate. The recommended dosage is 500 to 1,000 mg taken three times daily with meals.

- Guggulipid (5% guggulsterones) at 500 mg three times daily. This ayurvedic cure has been shown to significantly lower total cholesterol.

- Garlic at 600 to 900 mg daily. The total allicin content should be between 4,000 to 6,000 mcg. A review of 16 studies (952 people) found that garlic lowered total cholesterol levels by 12 percent after one to three months of treatment.

- Policosanol-an excellent supplement to lower total and LDL cholesterol. Take 10 to 20 mg at bedtime.

- A high-potency multivitamin or antioxidant formula. This will help keep cholesterol from being oxidized. Important antioxidants include vitamin C, E, selenium, CoQ10, alpha lipoic acid, and others.

LDL (Low-Density Lipoprotein)

Also referred to as "bad cholesterol," LDL is a type of lipoprotein that carries cholesterol from the liver to the blood vessel walls and body cells. Elevated levels are considered a major risk factor for the development of atherosclerosis and heart attack. Elevated LDL levels are even more of a concern if HDL levels are low. It is common for levels to increase in menopausal women.

Healthy value
- Below 130 mg/dl

Natural solutions
- Same as for total cholesterol. Antioxidant supplements are even more important if LDL is elevated.

HDL (High-Density Lipoprotein)

Often referred to as "good cholesterol," HDL works to transport cholesterol from the artery walls to the liver, as well as prevent some of the harmful effects of LDL. Good HDL levels are protective against heart disease. High levels of HDL help to offset some of the risk of elevated LDL levels.

Healthy value

❧ 50 mg/dl or higher

Natural solutions

❧ Same program as for total cholesterol and LDL.

❧ Exercise to increase HDL.

❧ Fish oil at 3,000 to 5,000 mg daily.

❧ L-carnitine at 1,500 to 3,000 mg daily.

❧ Chromium at 200 to 400 mcg daily.

Triglycerides

Triglycerides are fats in the blood that originate from the diet or are manufactured by the liver. People with diabetes and those who are overweight often have elevated triglyceride values. Elevated levels are associated with insulin resistance and coronary artery disease.

Healthy value

❧ Less than 150 mg/dl

Natural solutions

❧ Exercise.

❧ The same protocol as recommended for HDL.

❧ Pantethine at 300 mg three times daily.

Total Cholesterol / HDL

This ratio is used by doctors to estimate cardiovascular risk. Although there are many other important markers, this ratio is the most frequently calculated.

Healthy value

❧ Less than 4

Natural solutions

❧ Following the protocols for total cholesterol and HDL can improve this ratio.

~~~~~~

CHOLESTEROL WONDER

Policosanol is a dietary supplement derived from the outer wax of the sugar-cane plant or bees' wax. It is very effective at lowering elevated LDL and total cholesterol levels. Cholesterol-lowering effects are usually seen within the first six to eight weeks of use. According to a research review, a Policosanol dosage of 20 mg reduces LDL levels by 25–30 percent after six months of use, and HDL cholesterol increases by 15–25 percent after two months.

Studies have also proven Policosanol as effective as pharmaceutical "statin" cholesterol-lowering drugs, but without the side effects. One study of almost 28,000 showed that only 86 persons reported adverse effects, of which the most frequent was weight loss. Policosanol was also shown to reduce lipoprotein(a) levels significantly and to prevent LDL oxidation.

Lipoprotein(a) [also known as Lp(a)]

Lp(a) seems to play a role in blood-clot formation. Elevated levels of this lipoprotein, which contains an LDL molecule, are considered a stronger risk factor for heart problems than elevated LDL. As genetics appear to play a large role in raising Lp(a), a family history of heart disease makes testing for this marker especially important.

Seemingly healthy persons who have "normal" cholesterol levels, abstain from unhealthy lifestyle practices (such as smoking and high-fat diets), exercise, and have normal blood pressure may still be prone to a heart attack because of elevated Lp(a). Perhaps that's why several studies have shown elevated Lp(a) to be one of the best predictors of coronary artery disease. One must also remember that widely used cholesterol drugs such as Mevacor® and Zocor® do not lower Lp(a) levels, but may, in fact, increase it! On the other hand, some studies have shown that estrogen replacement decreases Lp(a).

Healthy value
&. Less than 32 mg/dl

Natural solutions

- ✒ Niacin (inositol hexaniacinate) at 500 to 1,000 mg three times daily with meals.

- ✒ Coenzyme Q10 soft gel at 100 to 200 mg daily.

- ✒ Policosanol 10 to 20 mg before bedtime.

Homocysteine

This byproduct of protein metabolism has been shown to be a major risk factor for cardiovascular disease. Studies on women have shown it to be an independent risk factor for heart attacks.

Elevated levels of homocysteine result from the body's inability to metabolize the amino acid methionine effectively. Elevations of homocysteine are also associated with birth defects, Alzheimer's disease, rheumatoid arthritis, multiple sclerosis, and osteoporosis. For approximately 5 to 10 percent of the population, elevated levels are due to genetics. For others, a diet low in B vitamins hinders the body's ability to process homocysteine. For both scenarios, supplementation with vitamin B12, folic acid, and B6 can work wonders to bring toxic homocysteine levels into the normal range. However, the dosage varies depending on the individual. You will need to work with a doctor to find out what levels of these B vitamins are needed to bring down your levels if they are elevated. This will require lab testing.

Healthy value

- ✒ 10 μol/L or less

Natural solutions

- ✒ B12 at 800 mcg to 2 mg. (Your doctor will help you determine this.)

- ✒ Folic acid at 1 to 10 mg. (Your doctor will help you determine this.)

- ✒ B6 at 20 to 100 mg. (Your doctor will help you determine this.)

&- Trimethylglycine (TMG) at 500 to 1,000 mg daily.

&- S'Adenosylmethionine (SAMe) at 200 to 400 mg daily.

NOTE: Dietary supplements designed to lower homocysteine levels are available. They usually contain B12, folic acid, B6, and sometimes TMG all in one formula so that you do not have to purchase them separately.

C-Reactive Protein

This is a marker for a chronic, low-grade inflammation that sometimes occurs in the blood vessels.

Measuring high-sensitivity C-reactive protein (hs-CRP) allows doctors to detect cardiovascular risk even among healthy people with no symptoms or other risk factors. C-reactive protein is a completely separate risk factor from the other cardiovascular markers, with elevated levels increasing a person's risk of cardiovascular disease from about two- to nearly fivefold. The Women's Health Study found that hs-CRP was "the single strongest predictor of risk" in women. It proved an even better predictor than LDL cholesterol.

It is thought that this protein disrupts fatty plaque build-up inside blood vessels, resulting in blood clots that trigger a heart attack, stroke, or other cardiovascular event. CRP also shows the ability to bind with LDL and make it more likely to adhere to artery walls, as well as cause LDL to oxidize. Previous infections may be involved with the initial triggering of the chronic inflammation that is detected by C-reactive protein. One study found that postmenopausal hormone replacement increased the levels of C-reactive protein two times higher on average than women not on hormone replacement.

Healthy value

&- Less than 1.69 mg/L

Natural solutions

&- Exercise, smoking cessation, weight loss, and improved glycemic regulation and blood pressure control may help to reduce inflammation and lower levels.

&- Vitamin E at 800 IU daily.

- Bromelain at 1,500 mg daily.
- Fish oil at 3,000 to 6,000 mg daily.
- GLA at 100 to 200 mg daily.
- MSM at 2,000 to 5,000 mg daily.

Fibrinogen

Fibrinogen is a substance that plays a role in the clotting process. Elevated levels lead to increased blood clots and "thickening" or increased viscosity of the blood. Fibrinogen is also an independent cardiac risk marker. Higher levels occur in people with cardiovascular disease and in those at risk because of smoking, obesity, lipid imbalances, and diabetes.

The Framingham Offspring Study measured fibrinogen in over 2,600 adults of an average age of about 55 years. Similar results were found as in previous studies, which associated high fibrinogen levels with a sixfold greater risk of developing coronary disease when combined with high LDL cholesterol, and a threefold greater independent risk of suffering a coronary event in patients with angina.

Healthy value

- Between 180 and 300 mg/dl

Natural solutions

- Smoking cessation.
- Bromelain at 1,500 to 3,000 mg daily.
- Fish oil at 5,000 to 7,000 mg daily.
- Vitamin E at 800 to 1,200 IU daily.
- Ginger root at 1,500 mg daily.
- Garlic at 600 to 900 mg daily. The total allicin content should be between 4,000 and 6,000 mcg.

Apolipoprotein A-1 (APO A-1)

This is a component of HDL and is associated with a protective effect against cardiovascular disease. Its value usually correlates with the HDL level.

Apolipoprotein B

This is a component of LDL. High levels are also associated with an increased risk of cardiovascular risk.

Apo B / Apo A-1 ratio

This is an important ratio used to evaluate cardiovascular risk.

NONDIRECT MARKERS

The following are what I call nondirect markers of cardiovascular risk. They are not considered direct tests of heart disease risk, but they can be significant contributing factors if they're out of balance.

Iron

Researchers are concerned that too much iron in the body leads to increased free-radical levels and oxidative damage of LDL cholesterol. This is one reason why I don't recommend that women supplement with iron unless they have had a blood test that determines they are anemic because of iron deficiency. However, the bigger concern is for people who have a genetic condition known as hemochromatosis, where intestinal iron absorption is greatly increased and a toxic build-up occurs. Many people are unaware they have this condition, and as a result their risk of heart disease may be elevated.

Blood tests can determine iron levels. Ferritin levels—the storage form of iron—should be measured, as should transferring saturation and total iron-binding capacity. Testing is also available for the other heavy metals such as lead, mercury, and cadmium.

Natural solutions

- ❧ Have your physician do screening tests for your iron levels. For those diagnosed with hemochromatosis, the standard treatment is to periodically draw blood.

Insulin resistance

People who consume diets high in refined carbohydrates and have low exercise activity, combined with nutritional deficiencies and a genetic susceptibility, often find themselves battling insulin resistance, which can be a major factor in heart disease. Excessive levels of insulin promote oxidation of cholesterol and thus plaque formation on the artery walls. They can also make the blood vessels more rigid. It is well known that those who have diabetes are at a much-increased risk for cardiovascular disease.

Many experts consider insulin resistance the immediate precursor of diabetes. As with diabetes, the condition leads to increased triglycerides and decreased HDL, as well as high blood pressure. Insulin and blood-sugar levels can and should be tested by your doctor as part of a comprehensive screening.

People diagnosed with heart disease, or those trying to lose weight, often make the mistake of eating a low-fat diet and increasing their carbohydrate intake. For some people this can lead to disaster because excessive carbohydrate intake (often of simple sugars like white breads, pastas, and so on) can lead to elevated blood-sugar levels and increased insulin levels. As a result, insulin levels spike, body fat is stored, and the promotion of arteriosclerosis occurs. A balanced diet with whole grains, vegetables, fruits, quality protein sources (fish, beans, lean poultry, nuts and seeds, and so on), and good fats will prevent insulin and blood-sugar problems. The key is to find what balance of carbohydrates, proteins, and fats works well for you.

Healthy value

- The "fasting insulin" level (measured when you haven't just eaten) should be somewhere between 4 to 15 μʊ/mol.

Natural solutions

- Healthful, low-carbohydrate diet.
- Chromium at 400 to 1,000 mcg daily.

&. Elemental vanadium at 100 to 200 mcg daily.

&. B-complex at 50 to 100 mg daily.

&. Magnesium at 500 mg daily.

POLYCYSTIC OVARY SYNDROME

Chronically high levels of insulin can significantly increase the heart-attack risk for women with polycystic ovary syndrome (PCOS), a sex-hormone disorder that affects as many as one out of every 15 premenopausal women. The condition often causes facial and body hair growth, lack of ovulation, and infertility. Researchers at the University of Calgary evaluated metabolic and cardiovascular risk parameters in 57 women with PCOS. They found that 75 percent of them had high levels of insulin, and that "cardiovascular risk factors [were] up to five times as prevalent" in this group as compared with PCOS patients who had normal insulin levels.

High blood pressure

Hypertension is one of the most significant risk factors for heart disease. When the pressure inside the blood vessel walls is too great, LDL cholesterol is deposited on the artery walls and plaques form. This predisposes you to heart attack, heart failure, and stroke. Approximately 23 percent of the female adult population have hypertension—an alarming figure.

Healthy value

&. An optimal blood pressure reading is 120/80 or less.

&. Systolic blood pressures 140 and higher, and diastolic readings of 90 or higher are considered to be hypertension. The Nurses' Health Study found that women between the ages of 35 and 65 with a high blood pressure have a risk of coronary artery disease three and a half times that of women with normal blood pressure.

Natural solutions

- Weight management through healthful diet and exercise.
- Stress reduction.
- Mineral balance (such as calcium, potassium, and magnesium).
- Adequate water intake.
- Coenzyme Q10 at 100 mg daily.
- Hawthorne Berry at 300 mg 3 times daily.

Hormone balance can also be a factor in hypertension. For a more detailed natural approach, see Chapter 12.

Smoking

You know that smoking is a deadly habit. Beyond the fact that it is the leading cause of lung cancer, smoking has been shown in studies to increase the risk of coronary artery disease from three to six times normal. The risk is even deadlier when a woman taking birth-control pills smokes. So my recommendation to quit smoking is obvious. As a matter of fact, I would recommend that if you smoke, your first order of business should be to stop. Work with a holistic doctor or support group to help you get through the initial withdrawal stage.

Antioxidant status

Your body is designed to protect itself against the damaging effects of oxidation. How effective it is in doing so depends on your intake of antioxidants in food. Current research is showing the beneficial effect of supplemental antioxidants in helping to prevent heart disease and other chronic illness. Tests are available that can measure the levels of many of these antioxidants as well as the level of oxidative stress occurring in your body.

Stress

Your ability to handle stress and incorporate stress-reducing techniques on a regular basis is one of the most fundamental techniques of living a long, healthy life free of cardiovascular and other diseases. Quite often the problem is not the stress itself but how we perceive it. High, prolonged levels of perceived stress can lead to conditions such as angina or heart attacks because they can cause the release of stress hormones such as cortisol and adrenaline, which over time can lead to a breakdown of the cardiovascular and immune systems.

Natural solutions

- Exercise.
- Prayer.
- Quiet time.
- Pets.

LAUGH YOUR WAY TO HEALTH

Researchers from the University of Maryland School of Medicine have found that laughter and a good sense of humor may actually provide some degree of protection against heart disease. Researchers evaluated the responses of 300 people to potentially humorous situations. Half of these individuals had experienced a previous heart attack or other indicator of heart disease, while the other 150 were healthy. By questionnaire, both groups indicated how they would respond to specific scenarios that could cause a stress response (a major risk factor for heart disease) such as arriving at a party dressed in clothing identical to one of the other guest's, or having a drink accidentally spilled on them by a waiter while dining with friends. Those with the highest "humor scores" had a 48-percent lower risk of heart disease, independent of their age or sex. By contrast, people with heart disease were much less likely to use humor as an adaptive mechanism. It is thought that laughter helps to reduce the effects of stress and prevent the inflammatory triggers that lead to artery inflammation and damage, as well as relax the lining of the blood vessels.

Depression

Studies have shown that people who suffer from depression have a greatly increased risk for heart disease. Depression has been shown to be a major determinant of cardiac death in those with or without symptomatic heart disease.

So what do you do if depression is a problem? Your best bet is to work with a healthcare professional and a minister of your "faith" to figure out why it is a problem. Here are some common reasons:

- Loneliness
- Grief
- Suppressed grief, anger, or emotions
- Suffering with a chronic disease or recovering from heart surgery
- Nutritional deficiencies
- Hormone and biochemical imbalances
- Side effects of medications

Natural supplements such as St. John's Wort, Ginkgo biloba, and SAMe can be of great supportive value for those with mild to moderate depression. Work with a holistic doctor to determine the optimal program for you.

Exercise

It is well known that physically active women have lower rates of coronary artery disease than sedentary women. Since Chapter 8 describes exercise and its benefits in detail, I say here only that recent research has shown less-than-vigorous exercise lowers the risk of heart disease. One large study found that at least one hour of walking per week predicted a lower risk of heart disease. This was true for women at high risk for heart disease, including those who were overweight, had increased cholesterol levels, or were smokers.

Weight

Tied strongly with the concepts of insulin resistance, diet, genetics, and exercise is weight. Being overweight places more stress on the heart, increases the likelihood of heart disease, causes high blood pressure, and elevates triglycerides. I find that people lose weight most successfully with a multipoint approach involving diet, exercise, emotions, hormone balancing, and nutritional supplements.

Age

Advancing age is often mentioned as a risk factor for heart disease, but statistically speaking, one can make the same categorization for most chronic diseases. Besides, why compare yourself to the average American your age when her lifestyle choices were probably not so healthy as they should have been. If you pay attention to your diet, lifestyle, and have a knowledgeable physician work with you on monitoring your cardiac health, age should not be a risk factor.

Dr. Tori Hudson, a highly respected expert in women's health, poignantly states in her book *Women's Encyclopedia of Natural Medicine,* "If one looks at the CAD (coronary artery disease) death rate for women, from birth to age 90, one finds it steadily increasing. In other words, it does not rise any faster after menopause than before." She then goes on to state, "This erroneous view is the foundation of why conventional hormone replacement therapy is recommended to virtually every woman after menopause."

Genetics

Certainly genetics can play a role in your risk of heart disease, but even though you have no control over which genes were passed onto you, you can alter the way they are expressed in your life. For example, elevated homocysteine, a condition caused by genetic predisposition, can be reduced with B vitamins. Niacin can reduce Lp(a). A diet rich in vegetables, fruits, and whole grains can lower cholesterol. Exercise can reduce cholesterol and improve the good HDL cholesterol. Stress reduction and smoking cessation obviously play major roles in how your genetic susceptibility will effect your life. All in all, genetics are only one factor among many that influence your cardiac health.

DO YOU NEED HORMONES TO PREVENT HEART DISEASE?

I have saved the issue of hormone replacement therapy (HRT) and heart disease until now so that you could first consider the many other factors that influence your risk for heart disease, and discover that there are many effective, nontoxic natural approaches to combat and reduce that risk.

With that said, the question of HRT's effectiveness in preventing heart disease remains. Unfortunately, there is no clear answer. My view is that HRT should not be recommended as a general therapy for women, as it currently is. However, in specific cases, HRT may be indicated as part of a comprehensive approach to prevent heart disease.

NOT ENDORSED BY THE FDA

It is interesting to note that the Food and Drug Administration (FDA) has never approved or endorsed the use of hormone replacement for preventing heart disease in women. Why not? My educated guess is that too many studies of HRT and heart disease are in conflict with each other. The FDA needs clear, unequivocal proof of the effectiveness of HRT for this use, and, so far, none has been forthcoming. The FDA has approved the use of HRT only for relieving menopausal symptoms such as hot flashes, and so on.

BENEFICIAL EFFECTS OF ESTROGEN ON CARDIOVASCULAR RISK MARKERS

It is well documented that estrogen replacement has benefits on many risk markers of cardiovascular disease. These include:

- Total cholesterol, low-density lipoprotein cholesterol, apolipoprotein B, and lipoprotein(a) levels
- High-density lipoprotein cholesterol level
- Homocysteine level
- Fibrinogen level
- Plasminogen activator inhibitor-1 (improved fibrinolysis)
- Insulin sensitivity
- Arterial wall flexibility

NOTE: Synthetic estrogen has been shown to increase C-reactive protein, which increases cardiovascular risk.

HOW EFFECTIVE IS ESTROGEN REPLACEMENT?

Several observational studies are often cited as demonstrating that hormone replacement therapy (HRT) reduces the risk of a heart attack by approximately 40–50 percent. At first glance this seems like a substantial benefit for women who use HRT. However, a commentary in the medical journal *Postgraduate Medicine* warns, "These observational data must be interpreted with caution. Patients who take estrogen may be more likely than other women to exercise, eat a low-fat diet, and live a healthy lifestyle. These factors are difficult to account for in observational studies."

In fact, it is generally agreed upon that women who take estrogen are healthier to start with than non-estrogen users. They also tend to be leaner, to be of higher socioeconomic status, to have better access to healthcare, and to visit their doctor more frequently.

The fact is heart disease was much less prevalent before estrogen replacement was ever introduced in this country. Due to refined foods, smoking, increase in obesity and diabetes, lack of physical activity, and other non-hormonal factors, the incidence of heart disease has greatly increased since the 1930s. Although estrogen replacement has benefits for menotype-C women during menopause, there is no direct evidence that low estrogen levels are a direct cause of heart disease.

As you can see, estrogen does have many benefits on cardiovascular risk markers. It also seems to have some antioxidant effect. But as you know, diet, lifestyle changes, and nutritional and herbal supplements can all lower these risk factors as or more effectively. The obvious advantage with the natural approach is that the increased risk of breast and endometrial cancer, as well as blood clots, gallbladder disease, and other potential side effects, is not a concern.

This book is all about creating a personal, tailor-made approach to your individual menopause experience. The same principle applies to your use of hormone replacement for the prevention of heart disease. If you are menotype C, you are going to be on hormone replacement. In certain menotype A and B cases, the use of hormone replacement may also be considered. For example, let's say a meno-type A or B woman has a significant elevation of lipoprotein(a) and/or other risk factors. Then estrogen replacement is a consideration. Of course, I prefer natural hormone replacement. Although natural hormones have not been studied for heart disease as synthetic estrogen has, many practitioners, including myself, have seen it improve cardiovascular risk markers.

HEART-HEALTHY DIET

Eating unrefined, whole grains; fresh vegetables and fruit; and cold-water fish such as salmon all contribute to a healthy cardiovascular system. Extra-virgin olive oil and flaxseed oils should be your choices for cooking. Avoid high intake of simple sugars and processed flours, red meat, dairy products, and especially cut down on fried foods, which contain harmful trans-fatty acids. Use cardiovascular-friendly spices in your cooking such as basil, rosemary, oregano, and garlic.

Don't underestimate the power of a healthy diet on the heart. Dr. Dean Ornish has shown in studies that a vegetarian diet, along with aerobic exercise, stress-management training, smoking cessation, and group psychosocial support, can actually reverse coronary artery disease. But you don't need to be a total vegetarian. The Mediterranean diet (abundant in plant foods such as vegetables, legumes, fruit, bread, pasta, and nuts, as well as olive oil, moderate amounts of fish, poultry, meat, dairy, eggs, and wine) has been shown to reduce the risk of a heart attack by as much as 70 percent.

HEART-HEALTHY SUPPLEMENTS

Most of these supplements have been described in Chapter 6, but let's just have a quick review.

- **Vitamin E** acts as an antioxidant to prevent the oxidation of LDL cholesterol. Also helps to lower C-reactive protein. Take a total of 400 to 800 IU daily.

WHEN HRT DOES MORE HARM THAN GOOD

A recently published study, the Heart and Estrogen/Progestin Replacement Study (HERS), has found that women who already had coronary artery disease who took synthetic estrogen and synthetic progesterone were not protected from heart attacks. The women in the group who took synthetic hormone replacement actually had a higher mortality rate in the first year as compared to women who took placebo! In addition, the group receiving hormones had three times more blood clot events and 40 percent more cases of gallbladder disease.

C-reactive protein, one of the most important risk markers for heart disease, has been shown to increase with the use of synthetic estrogen, and the simultaneous use of synthetic progesterone negates some of the beneficial effects estrogen has on cardiovascular risk factors.

- **Vitamin C** acts as an antioxidant. Take 500 to 1,000 mg daily as a preventive dosage.

- **Coenzyme Q10** is a specific nutrient required by the heart to contract strongly and regularly. Also acts as an antioxidant. For prevention of heart disease, take 30 to 50 mg daily. For those who already have heart disease, 100 to 300 mg daily is recommended.

- **L-Carnitine** helps the heart "burn" fat for fuel. Excellent for persons with high triglycerides and angina. Take 250 to 500 mg daily for prevention; take 1,500 to 3,000 mg daily if you already have cardiovascular disease.

- **Magnesium** is a mineral required for energy production and heart contraction. An average dosage is 500 mg daily.

- **B vitamins** reduce homocysteine build-up. A 50- or 100-mg complex daily is used for preventive purposes.

- **Essential fatty acids:** A daily dose of 3,000 mg of fish oil is a good preventive.

NOTE: Formulas are available that contain many of the major antioxidants. They are useful in addition to a high-potency multivitamin.

SHE TRIED IT

Sue, a very motivated 50-year-old menotype-C patient, came to see me three years ago. She had been on synthetic hormones from her doctor for the relief of hot flashes. She had recently taken herself off hormone replacement because she was concerned about developing breast cancer. Since she had not had bloodwork done in a long time, I ordered a blood screen that included a check for cardiovascular markers. The test showed a dangerously high cholesterol level of 395, triglycerides of 290, and low HDLs. Her thyroid was normal. The first step in her menotype program was to change her diet by increasing her vegetables and whole grains, staying away from fried foods, increasing her intake of fish and poultry, and drinking more water. For supplements, she began taking guggulipid, 100 mg of B complex, 800 IU of vitamin E, and a multivitamin. Sue increased her exercise by walking three times a week. Within three months, her cholesterol was down to 190 and the rest of the markers were in the normal range.

.

11

$\mathcal{B}$ONES OF STEEL

$\mathcal{O}$steoporosis is a concern for all menotypes, but menotype C's (especially those who have had their ovaries removed) and some menotype B's need to pay particular attention to the problem, since these two menotypes are susceptible to hormone deficiencies that can accelerate bone loss.

WHAT IS OSTEOPOROSIS?

Osteoporosis or "porous bone" is a disease that deteriorates bone tissue. It is often referred to as a "silent disease" since bone loss may occur without symptoms, eventually making the bones very fragile and more likely to fracture. I have seen many patients with osteoporosis suffer a fracture by simply bumping into something or taking a mild fall. In severe cases, you can develop collapsed vertebrae while just sitting down. Collapsed vertebrae generally result in back pain, loss of height, or stooped posture.

AN ALL-TOO-COMMON CONDITION

According to the National Osteoporosis Foundation, 8 million American women and 2 million men have osteoporosis, and millions more have low bone density. This number grows daily as the population ages. Some more sobering statistics from the Foundation on osteoporosis:

❧ One in two women and one in eight men over age 50 will have an osteoporosis-related fracture in their lifetime.

❧ One and a half million fractures occur each year as the result of osteoporosis. This includes these most common fracture sites: 300,000 hip fractures; 700,000 vertebral fractures; 250,000 wrist fractures; and 300,000 fractures at other sites.

The financial medical costs due to osteoporosis and associated fractures in the U.S. are staggering, with well over $38 million daily and still rising!

The most serious fact is that 12 to 20 percent of women with osteoporosis who suffer a hip fracture die from complications. In addition, as high as 25 percent of those who survive the hip fractures require long-term care in a facility for a year after the fracture.

THE IMPORTANCE OF STRONG BONES

A recent survey of over 200 women aged 75 years and older revealed that 80 percent would rather be dead than experience the loss of independence and quality of life resulting from a bad hip fracture and subsequent admission to a nursing home.

SIMPLIFIED BONE ANATOMY

There are two types of bone: trabecular and cortical. *Trabecular* bone is spongy and located inside the bone where the bone marrow is. It is concentrated in the vertebrae (80-percent trabecular and 20-percent cortical) and makes up 50 percent of the pelvis. It is also concentrated in the ribs and jaw. Trabecular bone is much more porous and metabolically active than cortical bone, and more susceptible to bone loss. Its strength is greatly influenced by hormones (especially low levels of estrogen), immobilization, and the use of certain steroid medications (such as prednisone).

Cortical bone is the hard, protective covering of bone you find in the long bones of the arms and legs. Its strength is greatly influenced by mineral intake (that is, calcium).

Collagen is an important protein that works to provide reinforcement to connective tissue such as bones so that they are less likely to break yet remain flexible. Collagen also allows minerals and other important protein substances to bind together to form bone.

A LIVING TISSUE

You may think of bone as a solid structure that gives us our shape and allows us to move. However, like the rest of our body, bone is a living tissue that is constantly remodeling itself by breaking down and reforming. There are two groups of specialized cells in the bone that are involved with bone remodeling: osteoclasts, which break down bone, and osteoblasts, which build bone. Diet, exercise, hormone activity, and other factors affect the activity of osteoclasts and osteoblasts. For example, exercise stimulates osteoblast activity while smoking increases osteoclast activity.

The key to maintaining good bone density is to create more bone than you lose.

MANY FACTORS TO CONSIDER

There are many risk factors for osteoporosis. Other than undergoing a bone-density study, the best way to analyze your risk is to assess yourself with the following summary of risk factors. Some, such as genetics and race, you cannot control, but most you can, including diet, lifestyle habits (such as smoking and alcohol), hormone balance, exercise, and choice of medications. Go through this list and circle the risk factors that pertain to you.

- Gender: female
- Age: increases as one ages, especially postmenopausal

- Ethnicity: Caucasian or Asian

- Family history of osteoporosis

- Never pregnant (full-term pregnancy)

- History of stress fractures

- Premature menopause

- History of amenorrhea (no menstrual periods, not including when pregnant), anovulation (not ovulating regularly), menses start late in life, and infrequent menses

- Thin or small body frame and low body fat

- Medical conditions (for example, diabetes, Cushing's disease, anorexia nervosa, bulimia, kidney and liver disease, homocysteinemia)

- Medications (such as anticonvulsants, prednisone, heparin, methotrexate, lithium, isoniazid, furosemide, antacids, chemotherapy, thyroid hormone [too much])

- Diet high in: caffeine, alcohol, sugar, phosphate (soda), sodium, animal protein

- Surgeries: complete thyroid removal, surgical resection of the stomach or small intestine

- Malabsorption (poor absorption of food)

- Lack of sun exposure (vitamin D from sun)

- Smoking

- Inactivity

- Hormone connection

THE ROLE OF ESTROGEN
(AND OTHER HORMONES)

It is generally accepted that the declining levels of estrogen during and after menopause are a contributing factor to bone loss in women. Estrogen therapy can reduce the loss of bone and, in some cases, increase bone density. It also reduces the risk of fractures in women with osteoporosis by approximately 50 percent. However, if the estrogen therapy is discontinued, bone-protective effects are lost. Many women either refuse synthetic estrogen replacement or stop using it because they're afraid of breast and uterine cancer.

Natural hormone replacement makes more sense, as it doesn't carry the same risks as the synthetics. For the prevention and treatment of osteoporosis, natural progesterone is generally used either by itself or in addition to bioidentical estrogen. While little scientific literature exists on the effectiveness of these natural substances in preventing bone loss, many holistic doctors report benefits among patients who use them.

Testosterone is an important hormone for bone health, and some studies have shown it benefits women with osteoporosis. As with any hormone, it needs to be well monitored.

Growth hormone is being taken more seriously as a therapy for osteoporosis, as it appears to stimulate bone growth. While research is ongoing, it should be considered for more serious cases of osteoporosis.

Too much thyroid hormone from a hyperfunctioning thyroid gland (hyperthyroidism) or from too high of a dosage of thyroid medication can accelerate bone breakdown and lead to osteoporosis. This is why anyone on thyroid medication needs to be monitored.

Parathyroid hormone (PTH), secreted by the parathyroid glands, which are located on the back sides of the thyroid, is released when blood levels of calcium are too low. The body needs to maintain a narrow range of blood calcium and part of PTH's action is to increase bone breakdown to free up calcium from the bones.

Calcitonin is a hormone secreted by the thyroid in response to elevated blood levels of calcium. This hormone stimulates the osteoblasts to use calcium to build more bone and decreases osteoclast activity.

IMMUNE SYSTEM CONNECTION

Researchers have found that an imbalanced immune system can contribute to osteoporosis. Specifically, a group of immune system cells known as cytokines (of which there are various types) can either hasten bone loss or stimulate bone growth. Certain cytokines initiate a type of autoimmune response whereby the immune system attacks its own tissues. This type of inflammatory reaction can lead to bone breakdown. Fortunately, a healthy diet, nutritional supplements, stress-reduction techniques, and hormone balance contribute to normal cytokine activity.

MEASURING YOUR BONE DENSITY

The only sure way to know the status of your bone density is to have a specialized bone-density study. There are several ways to measure bone density, and fortunately all are painless. The "gold standard" is an x-ray known as dual energy x-ray absorptiometry (DEXA). This is a low-dose x-ray of the lower spine and hip. Your report will compare your bone density with that of a healthy young, female adult and with that of a typical woman your age. This measurement is used in deciding whether hormone replacement is indicated for you. You have a mild risk for fracture if your bone density is 75%–85% of that of a young adult, a moderate fracture risk at 65%–75%, moderate/severe at 55%–65%, and severe at less than 55% percent. For women with moderate to severe osteoporosis, the use of hormone replacement must be a strong consideration.

A newer bone-density test that is less expensive and easier to perform is the heel bone-density test. For this test, an ultrasound is used instead of x-ray. Since it is a mobile test and less expensive, it is increasing in popularity as a screening tool in health food stores, pharmacies, and shopping malls. If an abnormal result is found with this test, then a DEXA scan can be done for confirmation (although a DEXA is still better).

URINE TEST FOR BONE BREAKDOWN

A urine test that measures bone breakdown is becoming increasingly popular among nutrition-oriented doctors. When bone breaks down, it releases fragments of collagen into the urine. The two fragments most commonly measured are Pyridinium and Deoxypyridinium, which have proven excellent indicators of bone loss due to osteoporosis. This test is not a substitute for a bone-density test. After a bone-density test is done, ongoing urine tests can track bone turnover. If the level of these markers is too high, you may be breaking down too much bone. In this way you can assess how well your treatment/prevention program is working (for example, diet, exercise, supplements, hormones, and so on) and make changes as necessary.

COMMON PHARMACEUTICALS
FOR OSTEOPOROSIS

Although my personal belief is that natural supplements and changes in lifestyle work best for the prevention and treatment of osteoporosis, many conventional doctors want to put their patients on pharmaceutical drugs. To help you become a more educated patient and consumer, some of these drugs are listed below.

HRT

- **Premarin**® and other synthetic estrogen products by themselves or in combination with synthetic progesterone is the major conventional focus for the prevention and treatment of osteoporosis of postmenopausal women. Estrogen is most helpful in retarding bone loss when used early in menopause.

- **Fosamax**® **(Alendronate)** is a non-hormonal drug that has been shown to increase bone density and reduce the incidence of vertebral and hip fractures (*Physicians' Desk Reference,* 52nd edition [Montvale, NJ: Medical Economics Co., 1998, pp. 1658–1659]). It works by interfering with osteoclast activity so that bone breakdown decreases. It is mainly taken in tablet form but can also be given intravenously. The most common side effect of Fosamax® is irritation and ulceration of the esophagus. The drug must be taken upon arising in the morning at least one half hour before your first food, water, or medication of the day. It must also be taken with 6 to 8 ounces of plain water, and you must remain upright for at least 30 minutes after taking it.

- **Calcitonin (Micalcin)** is a hormone that works to stimulate bone formation and is used pharmaceutically as an injection, and more commonly as a nasal spray. Studies show that it increases bone density and reduces fracture risk. Nasal problems such as runny nose, bleeding nose, and drying of the nose are potential side effects. Back pain, arthritis, and headache are also possible, as are flushing and nausea.

- **Evista® (Raloxifene)** falls into the category of selective estrogen receptor modulators (SERM). It selectively stimulates estrogen receptors of the bone but not of the breast or uterine tissue. It has been shown to increase bone density and decrease spinal fractures. Hot flashes are one of the most common side effects. Many other designer SERMs for osteoporosis are on the horizon.

5 NATURAL WAYS TO BUILD BONES OF STEEL

No matter what your menotype or bone-density status, the following natural therapies work at removing the underlying cause(s) of osteoporosis and supply the building blocks or stimulus for bone formation.

1. Exercise

This is the no-brainer. Putting stress on your bones stimulates bone growth. The National Osteoporosis Foundation recommends the following exercises:

Walking	Weight-training
Stair stepping	Jogging
Hiking	Skiing
Dancing	Aerobics (low impact)

Work with an experienced trainer for a comprehensive program that includes resistance training.

2. Diet

One of the most powerful ways to prevent bone loss is through a healthy diet. The foods you eat can either build or destroy bone, and this is true for children as well as adults. Since bone is living tissue, it must be supplied with the proper nutrition to survive and thrive. What type of diet should you follow to ensure proper bone health? A balanced one. The following are tips to use in your mission to build bones of steel.

LOVE THOSE VEGETABLES. It is well known that a vegetarian diet is associated with a lower risk of osteoporosis and that vegetarians generally have a higher bone density later in life. This makes sense. Plants are full of nutrients, whereas animal protein increases calcium excretion. Many vegetables, especially the green ones, are valued by nutritionists for promoting alkalinity, which is also thought important for bone health. Sea vegetables are an excellent source of minerals, particularly calcium. Again, I am not promoting a vegetarian diet, but the bones benefit from your adding lots of vegetables to your diet.

ESSENTIAL FATTY ACIDS. Essential fatty acids such as you find in fish, flaxseeds, and some vegetable oils, as well as nuts such as walnuts, are important for bone health. They help to suppress the effects of inflammatory cytokines that contribute to bone breakdown. Animal studies have shown that they improve calcium absorption, reduce calcium excretion, and increase calcium deposition in the bones. You should consume essential fatty acids in your diet and in supplements to maintain your bone health.

PROTEIN BALANCE. Excessive animal protein is associated with increased risk for osteoporosis. This is another problem with the osteoporosis-promoting American diet. Eating too much animal protein may cause calcium loss as the body buffers the high acidity of animal protein with calcium. Try to increase the amount of vegetable protein (nuts, seeds, grains, legumes) in your diet as you decrease animal proteins (red meat, dairy products).

FATTY ACIDS: ESSENTIAL FOR BONES

A study of senior women (average age 79.5 years) looked at the effect of essential fatty acids on bone density. Women were given either a combination of calcium and essential fatty acids (DHA and GLA), or calcium and a placebo. Over the first 18 months, lower spine density remained the same throughout the treatment group, but decreased 3.2 percent overall in the placebo group. Thigh-bone density increased 1.3 percent in the treatment group, but decreased 2.1 percent in the placebo group. During the second period of 18 months with all patients receiving essential fatty acids, lower spine density increased 3.1 percent in patients who remained on active treatment, and 2.3 percent in patients who switched from placebo to active treatment. Thigh-bone density in the latter group showed an increase of 4.7 percent.

All of these numbers point to one conclusion: Essential fatty acids can help your bones to grow.

Moderate consumption of soy appears to be healthy for the bones. Soy phytoestrogens, called isoflavones, are thought to be the key to soy's protective effect on bone density. One recent *in vitro* study showed that soy extract encouraged bone formation by stimulating bone-building osteoblasts. Another recent study on perimenopausal women demonstrated that soy halts bone loss in the lumbar spine.

SUGAR. Refined sugar products make you excrete calcium in your urine. They also contribute to insulin resistance, which not only affects your heart and weight but also your bones.

REDUCE THE SODA. The occasional carbonated soft drink is fine but, when consumed in excess, contributes to osteoporosis. The phosphoric acid as well as the sugar cause you to excrete calcium in your urine. Plus some sodas contain caffeine. The popularity of these drinks among kids is alarming, as it's clearly putting an entire generation at increased risk for osteoporosis later in life.

CAFFEINE. Caffeine leads to urinary calcium excretion. If you are a coffee lover, then cut down to one to two cups a day, unless you already have osteoporosis in which case you should avoid coffee altogether. Green tea is an option (which contains significantly less caffeine) as are several other herbal beverages.

ALCOHOL. Excessive alcohol intake not only increases your risk of breast cancer and liver disease but also causes bone loss. A couple of glasses of wine a week is not a problem for your bones. Again, moderation is the key.

SODIUM. Excessive salt intake can take its toll on the bones by causing urinary calcium excretion. Pass on the salt shaker and be wary of canned and processed foods loaded with sodium.

THE COW'S MILK MYTH

Powerful media advertisement by the dairy industry has led people to believe that cow's milk is ambrosia to the bones. While dairy milk does contain approximately 300 mg of calcium per 8-ounce serving, the calcium is not all that well absorbed. Considering that milk is one of the most common food allergens (a problem for those with lactose intolerance), high in phosphorous (causes calcium excretion), and contaminated with hormones (unless organic), I do not recommend it as a primary source for calcium.

---

3. Stress Reduction

When the stress hormone cortisol is elevated for long periods of time, it leads to the breakdown of bone tissue. This is another reason why stress reduction (exercise, vacations, prayer, and so on) is so important.

4. Bone-specific Supplements

Following are your best bets in supplementation for maintaining good bone health.

CALCIUM. A study published in the *New England Journal of Medicine* stated that postmenopausal women who supplemented 1,000 mg of calcium daily experienced a 43-percent reduction in bone loss compared with women who weren't taking a calcium supplement. Unfortunately, most women do not consume enough calcium on a regular basis. The National Academy of Sciences recommends that women between the ages of 19 and 50 should consume 1,000 mg daily, and postmenopausal women consume 1,200 mg daily, but most women actually consume only about 600 mg a day.

Following is a listing of calcium content in food:

Wakame (sea vegetable), ½ cup, 1,700 mg

Agar (sea vegetable), ¼ cup, 1,000 mg

Nori (sea vegetable), ½ cup, 600 mg

Kombu (sea vegetable), ¼ cup, 500 mg

Sardines with bones, ½ cup, 500 mg

Tempeh, 1 cup, 340 mg

Collard greens, 1 cup, 355 mg

Cow's milk, 1 cup, 300 mg

Calcium-enriched Rice or Soy milk, 1 cup, 300 mg

Almonds, 1 cup, 300 mg

Spinach, 1 cup, 280 mg

Yogurt, 1 cup, 270 mg

Sesame seeds, ½ cup, 250 mg

Kale, 1 cup, 200 mg

Broccoli, 1 cup, 180 mg

Tofu, 1 cup, 150 mg

Walnuts, ¼ cup, 70 mg

Black beans, 1 cup, 60 mg

Lentils, 1 cup, 50 mg

If you take a calcium supplement, use a chelated form (generally bound to an amino acid) such as calcium citrate-malate, citrate, aspartate, or gluconate for improved absorption. Overall, calcium citrate-malate appears most easily absorbed, followed by citrate. Carbonate is low on the list. Calcium supplements are best taken with meals.

MAGNESIUM. Almost equal in its importance to calcium is the mineral magnesium. It is essential for proper calcium metabolism. You need it for parathyroid hormone production and release, which activates vitamin D, which in turn affects intestinal calcium absorption. Good food sources of magnesium include wild grain products such as brown rice, wheat bran, buckwheat, and rye. Other rich sources include kelp, almonds, tofu, and dark green vegetables. I recommend an average of 500 mg daily, although some patients with osteoporosis need to take higher dosages. Magnesium citrate or glycinate are good forms.

VITAMIN D. Vitamin D is an essential supplement for the prevention or treatment of osteoporosis. It works to improve intestinal calcium absorption and prevent the urinary excretion of calcium. Vitamin D is found in foods such as fish; fish liver oil (such as cod liver); butter; and fortified cereals, bread, and milk.

Sunlight initiates the formation of vitamin D in your skin, but this process appears to become less efficient as people grow older. In any case, many people don't get much sunlight. Some avoid the sun due to the fear of skin cancer, others live in a cold climate, and many just don't spend much time outdoors. One study looked at 249 healthy postmenopausal women, average age 61, each of whom took a daily calcium supplement to ensure that their intake, including food sources, totaled 800 mg. Half of the women received 400 IU of vitamin D and the other half placebos. Over the course of a year, the women receiving the additional vitamin D had a significant gain in bone density. Take 400 IU as a preventive dosage and 800 to 1,200 IU as a therapeutic dosage.

VITAMIN K. This vitamin helps form the protein osteocalcin, which attracts calcium into the bone matrix, and is important for the healing of fractures. Studies have shown that low vitamin K is associated with osteoporosis and fractures due to the disease. Vitamin K is found in green leafy vegetables such as Romaine lettuce, spinach, kale, and collard greens as well as broccoli, Brussels sprouts, and eggs.

Take a preventive supplemental dosage of 150 to 500 mcg daily. For those with osteoporosis, some nutritional doctors recommend 2 to 10 mg daily.

VITAMIN C. Good old vitamin C contributes to the formation of collagen, which is an integral component of bone formation. Vitamin C deficiency has been shown to cause osteoporosis in animal studies. Food sources include citrus fruit, broccoli, turnips, peppers, cauliflower, and potatoes.

I recommend 500 to 1,000 mg as a preventive dosage and 2,000 to 3,000 mg daily for those with osteoporosis.

SILICON. This mineral helps in the formation of collagen as well as other connective tissue. It also appears to be involved in calcification. It is found in unrefined grains such as oats and brown rice, as well as cucumbers, radishes, olives, white onions, and the herb Horsetail. Take 5 to 20 mg daily. Those who already have osteoporosis should work with their doctor to increase the daily dose of silicon.

BORON. Boron works to activate vitamin D, save magnesium, and increase estrogen for effective calcium metabolism. A 1988 study inspired great interest in demonstrating that boron supplementation reduced urinary calcium and magnesium excretion, and increased blood levels of estrogen (17-beta estradiol) by 44 percent. Food sources include fruits (such as apples and grapes), vegetables (such as broccoli and cabbage), and nuts. I recommend 3 to 5 mg daily.

ZINC. This mineral is required for many enzymatic reactions including bone formation and hormone synthesis (related to bone health). Zinc absorption often decreases as people age. Whole grains, legumes, nuts, and seeds are good sources. Take 15 to 30 mg daily. It is best taken apart from calcium supplements if possible. In addition, 2 to 3 mg of copper should be taken along with zinc to maintain a balance of the two minerals.

MANGANESE. Manganese is involved in calcification of bone. It is found in whole grains, nuts, meat, green leafy vegetables, and almonds. A good therapeutic dosage is 15 to 30 mg.

B VITAMINS. B12, folic acid, and B6 help to prevent the build-up of homocysteine, a byproduct of protein metabolism. High levels of homocysteine can interfere with bone formation. Take as directed in Chapter 10.

IPRIFLAVONE. This is a type of synthesized isoflavone that is similar to isoflavones found in soy. Several studies have proven it effective in maintaining and in some cases increasing bone density when combined with calcium, vitamin D, or hormone replacement. What is interesting about isoflavone is that it is able to act like estrogen with regard to its bone-health benefits, without any of the side effects estrogen carries. Ipriflavone stimulates osteoblasts to form fresh bone and decreases the activity of osteoclasts, the cells that break down bone. It also acts to enhance the bone-building action of calcitonin.

Several double-blind studies have shown that ipriflavone increases bone density when combined with calcium.

Ipriflavone also works well in combination with estrogen and may even allow for the use of lower doses of estrogen, reducing potential side effects.

The recommended dosage is 600 mg daily taken with food. I recommend it for women who have osteoporosis or those with a strong family history of the disease.

One negative study published in the *Journal of the American Medical Association* reported that ipriflavone combined with calcium was no better than placebo in slowing bone loss. In addition, 29 out of the 132 women taking ipriflavone developed a reduction in white blood cells, known as lymphocytes. Researchers have stated that this reduction in lymphocytes is not clinically significant. I have seen no problems with patients but still recommend periodic blood tests to make sure immune markers are normal. I remind doctors and consumers that over 60 studies have been done on ipriflavone with the majority quite positive with regard to bone health. Compared to the pharmaceutical options, ipriflavone is both effective and relatively safe.

DON'T FORGET DIGESTION. Strong digestion is important for the absorption of nutrients from food as well as the supplements women take. Studies have shown that approximately 40 percent of postmenopausal women have low stomach acid. Stomach acid is important for the absorption of minerals such as calcium. Chronic illness, stress, nutritional deficiencies, and certain medications can all lead to low stomach acid. Supplements such as betaine hydrochloric acid can be taken with meals to increase stomach-acid effectiveness, as can herbs such as Gentian Root.

One caution: These supplements should not be used if you have an active ulcer.

KEEP IT SIMPLE. How do you get all the vitamin and minerals you need plus ipriflavone? Simply take a high-potency multivitamin along with one of the many available "bone formulas." Take your two supplements with meals if digestion and absorption are an issue.

5. Natural Hormone Replacement

For all menotype C's and some menotype B's, estrogen, progesterone, DHEA, testosterone, and growth hormone (in some cases) are all indicated for an aggressive hormonal approach to halting and reversing this disease. Again, I prefer the natural versions of these hormones to their synthetic counterparts, even though there hasn't been much research on them.

Hormone testing as described in Chapter 4 is important to make sure you're receiving the right dosages of replacement hormones. In addition, the bone-resorption test described in this chapter, along with bone-density tests, can help you monitor the effectiveness of HRT therapy.

12

$\mathcal{N}$ATURAL SOLUTIONS TO COMMON FEMALE CONDITIONS

$\mathcal{A}$ woman will face many health challenges during her life. Some will appear only around or after her transition through menopause, others will show up sooner. Following is a list of common conditions and some advice on what to do about them.

ALZHEIMER'S DISEASE AND POOR MEMORY

Alzheimer's disease falls into a group of conditions known as dementia, which refers to a loss or worsening of memory and mental capacity. No one is yet certain what causes Alzheimer's disease. Stress, genetics, heavy metal accumulation (aluminum), oxidative damage, hormone imbalance (estrogen deficiency), a history of strokes, and nutritional deficiencies have all been proposed as possible culprits. While no cure exists, many researchers feel that Alzheimer's can be prevented through appropriate diet, lifestyle, and preventive medical approaches. Once Alzheimer's disease has begun, conventional or natural therapy may help to slow the progression of the disease.

Poor or declining memory during the menopausal transition can be related to hormonal changes as well as nutritional deficiencies and poor circulation to the brain. The natural therapies used for Alzheimer's are the same as those used for poor memory.

Nutrition

- *A diet high in plant foods* provides an abundant supply of antioxidants that prevent brain cell damage. Caffeine, sugar, and

215

artificial sweeteners should be avoided. Regular water consumption is important for brain hydration. Increase intake of cold-water fish, such as salmon, for the brain-healthy omega-3 fatty acids. Ground up flaxseeds and walnuts are also recommended.

NOTE: Smoking increases oxidative damage of brain cells and should be stopped.

Nutritional supplements

- *Phosphatidylserine (PS)* is a brain-specific phospholipid that has been most thoroughly researched with regard to its effect on Alzheimer's disease and may help slow progression. Also used for those with poor memory and concentration. Dosage is 300 mg daily.

- *Antioxidants* prevent oxidative damage of brain cells. Use an antioxidant formula or individual nutrients that contain vitamin C (1,000 to 2,000 mg), vitamin E (800 to 1,200 IU), CoQ10 (100 mg), selenium (200 mcg), mixed carotenoids (25,000 IU), and alpha lipoic acid (100 mg).

- *B12 and folic acid* will keep you from developing a deficiency that can mimic symptoms of Alzheimer's. Take 800 mcg to 1 mg of each daily.

- *Acetyl-L-carnitine* is a vitamin-like substance shown to be helpful for Alzheimer's and memory problems. Take 500 mg three times daily between meals.

- *Zinc* is important for proper brain function. Take 30 to 50 mg daily as part of a multivitamin or as a separate formula.

- *Essential fatty acids* are important components of the brain, which is composed of 60-percent fat. Take 300 to 500 mg of DHA or a blended formula.

- *Lecithin* provides acetylcholine, an important neurotransmitter that is deficient in Alzheimer's patients. Take 1,000 to 2,000 mg daily.

Herbal

❧ *Gingko Biloba* (24%) improves circulation to the brain and stimulates neurotransmitters involved with memory and concentration. Take 180 to 240 mg daily.

NOTE: High doses of Gingko Biloba should not be used if on blood-thinning medications.

❧ *Panax Ginseng* was historically used to revitalize the mind. Take 300 mg daily of a 4–7% ginsenoside extract.

Hormonal balancing

❧ Menotype B's may notice improvement with the use of natural progesterone and/or DHEA. Menotype C's may notice improvement with natural hormone replacement including DHEA, pregnenolone, estrogen, progesterone, and possibly testosterone.

ANXIETY

Millions of American women suffer from anxiety, which can cause feelings of nervousness or unease as well as shortness of breath, heart palpitations, and sweating. In more severe cases, panic attacks can occur. Worry, fear, and other stresses in life can be at the root of the problem. However, hormone and biochemical imbalances are common causes as well, as is often the case with women who have PMS or who are going through menopause. Synthetic hormones or improperly dosed hormones can bring on anxiety in some women. Low blood-sugar levels can also have this effect.

Nutrition

❧ *Avoid substances that can worsen anxiety,* such as caffeine, alcohol, and sugar. Regular meals or snacks should be consumed throughout the day to maintain even blood-sugar levels. Cold-water fish such as salmon, mackerel, halibut, and herring are helpful as they contain essential fatty acids, which can help reduce anxiety. Lastly, consume foods rich in calcium and magnesium, which help to relax the nervous system.

Nutritional supplements

- *Fish oil* increases essential fatty acids. Take 3,000 to 5,000 mg daily or one to two tablespoons of flaxseed daily.

- *Calcium and magnesium* work to relax the nervous system and muscles. Take 1,000 mg of calcium and 500 mg of magnesium daily.

- *B-complex* helps to counteract the effects of stress. Take a 100-mg B-complex daily.

Herbal

- *Kava* has been well studied for its ability to reduce anxiety and panic attacks. Take a product that contains 50 to 70 mg of kavalactones per capsule three times daily. Do not use in combination with pharmaceutical anti-anxiety medications, or alcohol and use on a short-term basis (4 weeks).

- *Passionflower* is a gentle yet effective nerve-relaxing botanical. Take 300 to 500 mg of the capsule form or 30 drops of the tincture three times daily.

- *Chamomile* is an excellent tea that can help relax the nervous system. Lemon Balm can be added for an even greater calming effect.

Homeopathy

- *Aconitum* is for acute anxiety attacks. Take two pellets of a 30C potency every ten minutes for up to three doses.

- *Rescue Remedy*™ is a homeopathic formula used to reduce anxiety and stress. Take five to ten drops as needed for anxiety.

Stress reduction

- The effects of stress can lead to anxiety. Exercise, prayer, counseling, and other stress-reducing activities are strongly recommended.

ARTHRITIS

Arthritis literally means inflammation of the joint. There are over 100 different types of arthritic conditions, with osteoarthritis (also known as degenerative joint disease) being the most common. Progression of osteoarthritis can begin by age 20, and is extremely common by age 70. Surveys have indicated that 80 percent of people over 50 have osteoarthritis. Under the age of 45, osteoarthritis is more common in men, but after that age it is ten times more common in women. This condition is characterized by the breakdown of the joints' cartilage (the part of the joint that cushions the bones). The breakdown of cartilage causes bones to rub against each other, resulting in pain and loss of movement. The hands and weight-bearing joints, especially the knees, hips, feet, and back, are most affected.

There are many factors that can cause and contribute to osteoarthritis: increasing age, obesity, history of joint injuries and trauma, genetic conditions, hormonal factors, nutritional deficiencies, and maldigestion to name a few.

Even your clothing can have an effect. Since osteoarthritis of the knee is twice as common in women as in men, researchers investigated the impact high-heeled shoes have on knee osteoarthritis. They concluded that the altered forces at the knee caused by walking in high heels may in fact predispose to degenerative changes in the joint.

As mentioned, the number of women affected by this disease increases greatly after the age of 45. This is the time most women are either perimenopausal or menopausal. Estrogen, progesterone, DHEA, and other hormones are declining. It is not clear how or why the declining levels of estrogen and progesterone affect joint pain, but it is clear that hormone balance is a key to prevent and treat osteoarthritis.

The association between synthetic hormone replacement therapy and a new diagnosis of arthritis has been examined by Canadian researchers. They found that women who used synthetic hormones for five years or longer were twice as likely as nonusers to develop osteoarthritis. An additional study examined the association of synthetic estrogen replacement therapy and the incidence of arthritis. Researchers found a 30-percent increased risk of arthritis among women who used this hormone for one to four years, and a 96-percent increased risk among those who used it for four to ten years. In other words, the longer they used synthetic hormones, the more likely they were to get arthritis.

Low thyroid function has also been implicated as a possible contributing cause of osteoarthritis.

Nutrition

- *A high-fiber, whole foods diet* is recommended.

- *Cold-water fish, walnuts, and flaxseeds* are important for their omega-3 fatty acid content. Omega-3 fatty acids help to reduce joint inflammation as well as lubricate the joints.

- *Avoid caffeine, alcohol, and sugar products.*

- *Wheat and dairy products* are common sensitivities that can cause flare-ups of osteoarthritis pain, so avoid them.

- *Avoid the nightshades.* Some people report benefit by giving up foods from the nightshade family (tomato, eggplant, potato, bell pepper).

Nutritional supplements

- *Glucosamine sulfate* can relieve arthritis pain and help rebuild cartilage. It can take four to eight weeks for noticeable improvement. Dosage is 1,500 mg daily.

- *MSM* is an excellent natural anti-inflammatory. Take 3,000 to 5,000 mg daily.

- *Essential fatty acid complex* reduces inflammation. Take in the form of fish oil (3,000 to 5,000 mg daily) or flaxseed oil (two tablespoons daily).

- *Vitamin C with bioflavonoids* protects against cartilage destruction. Take 2,000 to 3,000 mg daily.

❧ *Vitamin E* has natural anti-inflammatory effects. Take 800 IU daily.

❧ *Digestive enzymes* in a full-spectrum complex should be taken with each meal for improved food absorption and assimilation.

❧ *SAMe* can be used to reduce inflammation if other supplements are not helpful. (It is more expensive.) Take 600 to 800 mg daily.

Herbal

❧ *Bromelain* is a natural anti inflammatory. Take 500 mg three times daily between meals.

❧ *Boswellia* is another natural anti-inflammatory. Take 500 to 1,000 mg three times daily.

❧ *Black Cohosh* reduces joint and muscle pain as well as reduces such menopausal symptoms as hot flashes. Take 80 mg of a 2.5% triterpene glycoside.

Homeopathy

❧ *Rhus Toxicodendron* relieves any pain and stiffness that normally responds to movement and warm applications. Take two pellets of 30C potency twice daily for five days, and then as needed if you feel improvement.

Hormones

❧ *DHEA* is an option if testing shows low hormone levels. Average dosage ranges between 20 and 50 mg daily. Use under supervision of a doctor.

NOTE: Work with a doctor to make sure your hormones are balanced, especially estrogen, progesterone, and testosterone. If using synthetic hormone replacement, I suggest converting to natural hormone replacement.

CERVICAL DYSPLASIA

Cervical dysplasia refers to abnormal changes in the cells of the cervix that may lead to cervical cancer. A Pap smear can detect these changes. Most cases of cervical dysplasia (90 percent) are due to Human Papilloma Virus (HPV) infection, a sexually transmitted disease. It is estimated that close to 70 percent of women are infected with HPV at some point in their lifetime, but fortunately most do not develop dysplasia. Smoking also increases one's risk, as does having multiple sexual partners and having intercourse at an early age. While many cases of cervical dysplasia revert back to normal without any treatment, I recommend the implementation of a toxic-free naturopathic approach. More invasive and severe dysplasia requires surgical removal.

Natural medicine has a lot to offer in both the prevention and treatment of cervical dysplasia. Naturopathic physician Tori Hudson has led the way in researching natural treatments for this condition, and several studies confirmed that diet and nutritional supplements are effective against it.

Optimizing the immune system, which is responsible for fighting off viruses such as HPV, is one of the keys to treating cervical dysplasia. How do you do that? By improving your nutritional intake, reducing stress, and using immune-enhancing natural therapies as described here.

Nutrition

- *Increase your intake of fruits and vegetables* to seven to ten servings daily. They supply antioxidants and immune-enhancing phytonutrients that are needed for a healthy immune system and proper cell development. Leafy green vegetables are a good source of the B-vitamin folic acid, which is important in fighting this condition. Sugar products should be avoided, due to their suppressive effect on the immune system.

Nutritional supplements

- *Take a multivitamin without iron* every day.

• *Folic acid* can help. Therapeutic dosage is 5 to 10 mg daily. To maintain balance with other B vitamins, it should be taken along with a multivitamin or B-complex. For women with a history of abnormal Pap smears, 2 mg daily is a good preventive dosage.

NOTE: Recent studies have not found an association between the birth-control pill and cervical cancer, yet these pills do deplete B vitamins such as folic acid and B12, which are required for proper cell division. Therefore, women using the birth-control pill should supplement a 100-mg B-complex daily.

• *Vitamin C* supports the immune system and is effective for viral infections. I recommend 2,000 to 5,000 mg daily as a therapeutic dosage and 1,000 mg daily as a preventive dosage.

• *Selenium* is effective for chronic viral infections. Therapeutic dosage is 400 mcg daily, while 200 mcg is a good preventive dose.

• *Carotenoids* have an antioxidant effect and support the immune system. Take 150,000 IU daily as a therapeutic dosage and 25,000 IU for prevention.

NOTE: Skin can turn an orangish color on this high of a dosage, but the condition is harmless.

• *Vitamin A* is required for proper cell division and studies show women with cervical dysplasia have lower dietary intakes of vitamin A. It is best taken in a suppository for a localized effect and should be used under the guidance of a doctor.

Herbal

• Some of my favorite immunity-enhancing herbs are *Echinacea, Lomatium,* and *Astragalus.* Therapeutic dosage would be 30 drops or two capsules three times daily of any one of these herbs or a formula that contains a blend.

Homeopathy

ᐖ *Conium* is one of the more common remedies used for cervical dysplasia. Two pellets of 30C potency can be taken twice daily for 10 to 14 days. Otherwise, it is best to consult with a homeopathic practitioner for an individualized prescription.

Stress reduction

ᐖ The perceived effects of stress can hinder immune function, so exercise, prayer, counseling, and other stress-reducing activities are strongly recommended.

DEPRESSION

Depression is a common condition among women during the menopausal years. This can be due to hormonal changes, nutritional deficiencies, or emotional adjustment. Natural medicine can be quite effective in alleviating depression without the potential for toxic side effects that come with some pharmaceutical antidepressants. Of course, hormone balancing for one's menotype is important in treating depression associated with menopause.

Nutrition

ᐖ *Consuming regular meals that are not loaded with refined sugar products* is the first step in relieving depression. Blood-sugar balance is important for mood regulation, as the brain prefers to use glucose as its fuel.

ᐖ *Essential fatty acids,* particularly DHA (found in cold-water fish), are important for proper brain neurotransmitter balance. Cold-water fish such as salmon should be consumed three or more times weekly.

ᐖ *Flaxseeds* are recommended for their omega-3 content. Food sensitivities can also be involved with depression, and should be identified and treated.

Nutritional supplements

- *SAMe* has proven in excellent studies that it's useful in treating depression. It can be used in conjunction with pharmaceutical antidepressants with a doctor's supervision. I recommend a dosage of 600 to 800 mg daily.

- *5HTP* acts as a precursor to the neurotransmitter serotonin, which plays a role in mood regulation. Typical dosage is 200 to 300 mg daily.

NOTE: Do not use 5HTP if on pharmaceutical antidepressants.

- *B vitamins (folic acid, B6, B12, and other B vitamins)* can prevent depression that results from B-vitamin deficiencies. This type of depression becomes more of a problem as women age. Therapeutic dosages may need to exceed those in a multivitamin. Here's what you should be taking daily: Folic acid, 800 mcg; B6, 25 to 50 mg; and B12, 400 to 800 mcg.

- *Essential fatty acids* supply "good fats" required for brain health. Take a formula that includes at least 300 mg of DHA daily.

Herbal

- *St. John's Wort* is effective for mild to moderate depression. Women should take 300 mg two to three times daily of a standardized extract (0.3% hypericin and 3%–5% hyperforin).

NOTE: Do not use St. John's Wort if on pharmaceutical antidepressants.

- *Ginkgo Biloba* improves brain circulation and neurotransmitter action. Take 180 to 240 mg daily of a 24% flavoglycoside extract.

Homeopathy

- *Rescue Remedy*™ is a general remedy that can be useful in treating depression. Take 50 to 60 drops three times daily.

Hormonal

➤ *Natural hormones* can help. Some women experience depression as a side effect of the hormones they are taking, especially synthetic hormones such as Premarin® or Provera®. Menotype B's often have improvement using natural progesterone, while menotype C's often notice quick improvement when put on natural hormone replacement.

➤ *Have your thyroid tested,* as an underactive thyroid gland can also cause depression.

➤ *Have your hormones tested.* Low levels of other hormones, such as DHEA and testosterone, can also be a cause.

Stress reduction

➤ *Exercise* has been shown to be important in the treatment of depression.

➤ *Prayer* is also strongly recommended.

ENDOMETRIOSIS

Abnormal growths resembling tissue found in the endometrium (uterine lining) sometimes appear in locations other than the uterine lining. Common areas of occurrence include the ovaries and the pelvis.

This is a common condition, occurring in approximately 10 percent of all reproductive-age women. It is the most common gynecologic reason for women between the ages of 15 and 44 being hospitalized. Symptoms can include pain before or during the menses (and sometimes throughout the month), pain during intercourse, irregular cycles, and infertility. Other symptoms can include bloating, diarrhea, rectal bleeding with menses, pubic pain during urination, and low back pain. Diagnosis is done through biopsy.

Scientists have proposed several possible causes for endometriosis. These include heredity, retrograde menstrual flow, alteration of the immune system, and hormone imbalance. Conventional therapy focuses on pain-relieving medications, hormone therapy (birth-control pill and other hormone-altering drugs), and surgery. Interestingly, this condition usually improves or goes away after menopause.

Natural therapy can help by improving hormone balance through a healthful diet and liver detoxification. Some herbal and homeopathic medicines are also useful. Acupuncture can relieve the pain of endometriosis.

Nutrition

- *A high-fiber diet* is recommended as it promotes more efficient hormone metabolism. This includes vegetables, particularly cruciferous vegetables—such as broccoli, cauliflower, Brussels sprouts, and cabbage—that promote liver detoxification since they contain high amounts of the phytochemical Indole-3 carbinole.

- *Beets, artichokes, and carrots* are also good for liver detoxification.

- *Taking five to ten teaspoons of ground flaxseeds* daily is also recommended as the seeds contain hormone-balancing Lignans and omega-3 fatty acids that reduce inflammation.

- *Cultured yogurt* supplies friendly bacteria that help hormone metabolism.

- *Avoiding the wrong foods* can help. These include caffeine, alcohol, and sugar. Red meat and dairy products should be used sparingly, and must be organic and hormone free.

Nutritional supplements

- *Indole-3 carbinole* assists in the liver's detoxification of estrogen and other hormones. Take 300 mg daily.

- *D-glucarate* also assists in the liver's breaking down such hormones as estrogen. Take 500 to 1,500 mg daily.

- *Vitamin E* helps with hormone imbalance and inflammation. Take 800 IU daily.

🐾 *Essential fatty acids* reduce inflammation in the tissues. Take 4,000 mg of fish oil and 1,000 mg of evening primrose oil daily.

🐾 *High-potency multivitamins* contain B vitamins and other nutrients involved with hormone metabolism.

Herbal

🐾 *Vitex (Chasteberry)* can help balance estrogen and progesterone ratios. Take 40 to 80 drops of a standardized tincture or 240 mg of a 0.6% aucubin standardized capsule extract.

NOTE: Do not use Vitex (Chasteberry) along with birth-control pills.

🐾 *Milk Thistle* promotes liver detoxification. Take 200 mg of a 85% silymarin extract three times daily.

Homeopathy

🐾 *Caution:* Homeopathic remedies can be very effective for endometriosis but are best used under the guidance of a homeopathic practitioner.

Hormonal

🐾 *Natural progesterone* provides benefit for some women. It is best used under the guidance of a doctor as dosages differ depending on the woman. Some women require one-quarter teaspoon twice daily for three weeks on and then one week off during the menstrual flow. Other women do better by taking natural progesterone the week before the menstrual flow.

FIBROCYSTIC BREASTS

Fibrocysts are noncancerous lumps or cysts of the breasts that may or may not be painful. For many women, breast tenderness becomes noticeable prior to menstruation, indicating a hormonal cause. Thus, hormone balance through nutrition and natural therapy is a key to treating this condition.

Nutrition

᪥ *Avoiding caffeine* (coffee, soda, and chocolate) is important, as some studies, though not all, show it to be helpful. I find it makes a difference to some extent with most women who have this condition.

᪥ *A high-fiber diet* is recommended for hormone balance. This includes the use of ground-up flaxseeds (five to ten teaspoons daily).

᪥ *Essential fatty acid* balance is important. Cold-water fish, such as salmon, which are full of inflammation-reducing omega-3 fatty acids, should be part of your meal three times weekly.

᪥ *Olive oil* is also recommended. Use it on your salads.

᪥ *Reducing sugar intake* seems to help some women.

Nutritional supplements

᪥ *Vitamin E* reduces breast tenderness and the tendency to form cysts. Part of this benefit may come as the result of its role in estrogen metabolism. I have been impressed by the effectiveness of natural vitamin E for this condition. I recommend 800 to 1,200 IU daily for at least two months to see if it is helpful.

᪥ *Essential fatty acids* in fish oil (3,000 to 4,000 mg) or flaxseed oil (one to two tablespoons) along with the omega-6 fatty acid GLA (150 to 300 mg) as found in evening primrose oil, borage oil, or blended formulas, can be very helpful for this condition.

Herbal

᪥ *Vitex (Chasteberry)* works well after two or more cycles through its hormone-balancing effects. Take 40 to 80 drops of a standardized tincture, or 240 mg of a 0.6% aucubin standardized capsule extract.

NOTE: Do not use Vitex (Chasteberry) along with birth-control pills.

*❧ **Phytolacca Oil** has been historically used topically by naturo-pathic physicians and herbalists for breast cysts.

*❧ **Milk Thistle** promotes liver detoxification. Take 200 mg of 85% silymarin extract three times daily.

*❧ **Dandelion Root** also promotes liver detoxification. Take 300 mg three times daily with meals.

Hormonal

*❧ **Natural progesterone** can work very well for the relief of fi-brocystic breasts, but I reserve its use for more severe cases that are unresponsive to the other therapies listed. Typically, one-quarter teaspoon is applied to the breast tissue twice daily seven to ten days before the menses.

FIBROMYALGIA

This condition is characterized by achy pain, tenderness, and stiffness of muscles and soft tissues that you can reproduce by pressing specific trigger points. Fatigue, insomnia, depression, anxiety, and irritable bowel syndrome are common among those with fibromyalgia.

There can be many underlying causes for this condition, including hormone and neurotransmitter imbalances, nutritional deficiencies, poor digestive and detoxification functions, and reaction to stress. Some women experience the onset of fibromyalgia after an infection (such as mononucleosis or the flu), which suggests an autoimmune re-action. Others experience an onset after a car accident or physical in-jury. Many women can't identify an immediate cause.

Conventional therapy relies on treating symptoms with muscle relaxers and sleep medications. Natural therapy, on the other hand, can be quite effective in providing nontoxic, lasting relief of symptoms by addressing underlying causes.

Nutrition

- *Avoiding caffeine, alcohol, and sugar products* is important as these can worsen pain.

- *Identifying and treating food sensitivities* can be very helpful in relieving symptoms.

- *Omega-3 fatty acids* as found in flaxseeds and fish are important in coping with this disease.

- *At least six eight-ounce glasses of water* a day are recommended for detoxification. Penta® water is quite effective.

- *Supergreen foods* such as spirulina, alfalfa, wheatgrass, and chlorella promote detoxification which can be helpful.

Nutritional supplements

- *Magnesium* relaxes the nerves and muscles. Take 500 to 1,000 mg daily.

- *Calcium* also relaxes the nerves and muscles. Take 1,000 mg daily.

- *SAMe* has proven effective for this use in several studies. Start at a dosage of 800 to 1,200 mg daily.

- *5HTP* is a supplement that acts as a precursor to the neurotransmitter serotonin, and several studies show it beneficial for fibromyalgia. Typical dosage is 200 to 300 mg daily.

NOTE: Do not use 5HTP if on pharmaceutical antidepressants.

- *Digestive enzymes* improve digestion and absorption of food. Take two capsules of a full-spectrum digestive enzyme with each meal.

Herbal

- *St. John's Wort* improves serotonin balance, which results in better sleep, less depression and anxiety, and fewer symptoms of fibromyalgia. Women should take 300 mg two to three times daily of a standardized extract (0.3% hypericin and 3%–5% hyperforin).

NOTE: Do not use St. John's Wort if on pharmaceutical antide-pressants.

ᐟᐤ *Siberian Ginseng* helps reduce the effects of stress on the body. The dosage is 300 mg twice daily.

ᐟᐤ *Passionflower and Valerian* (30 drops of each) can be helpful a half hour before bedtime to promote sleep.

Homeopathy

ᐟᐤ *Caution:* I have found homeopathic medicines to be very help-ful, but they are best prescribed on an individual basis.

Hormonal

ᐟᐤ *Switching to natural hormones* is often beneficial in treating this condition, as synthetic hormone replacement worsens it for some women.

ᐟᐤ *Black Cohosh and natural progesterone cream* are both ef-fective in reducing fibromyalgia in perimenopausal women.

ᐟᐤ *Melatonin* can help improve insomnia, which is critical to treating this condition. Typical dose is 0.5 mg a half hour before bedtime.

ᐟᐤ *Thyroid* low thyroid is often involved. Work with a holistic doctor to improve thyroid function.

Lifestyle

ᐟᐤ *Acupuncture* can be helpful for pain relief and other symptoms associated with fibromyalgia.

GENITAL HERPES

Genital herpes is one of the most common sexually transmitted dis-eases in North America. An estimated one in five adults is believed to be infected with herpes simplex virus type 2 (HSV 2), the most com-mon cause of genital herpes. Herpes simplex type 1 (HSV 1), which is the virus that causes cold sores, can also cause genital herpes. The age of highest incidence in women is 20 to 24 years.

Genital herpes generally occurs in the genital and anal areas. Symptoms of initial infection usually occur four to seven days after contact. Primary infection is characterized by clusters of painful, superficial, red, raised lesions that turn into water-filled vesicles two to three days later. Ulceration and crusting then follow. Fatigue, body ache, nausea, swollen lymph nodes in the groin area, and headaches are also common during the initial outbreak.

Lesions that occur during the first outbreak are usually more severe and prolonged than those of recurrent outbreaks. Since outbreaks can occur without symptoms, it is imperative that "safe sex" is always practiced.

Zovirax® (acyclovir) and related antiviral drugs are commonly used to reduce the duration of acute infection and may help suppress future outbreaks. Nausea, vomiting, and headaches are the most common side effects.

The herpes virus remains dormant in the body under the surveillance of the immune system. Thus, any factor that compromises the immune system (nutrition, stress, and so on) can make you more vulnerable to an outbreak.

Genital herpes is considered incurable, although I have worked with patients who have not had recurring outbreaks after natural therapy.

Nutrition

ᵛ *Avoid foods that contain large amounts of the amino acid arginine* (especially during times of outbreak). Arginine is used by the herpes virus to replicate itself. Foods that are high in arginine include chocolate, peanuts, almonds, cashews, and sunflower seeds.

ᵛ *Lysine,* another amino acid, can be helpful in the inhibition of herpes virus replication. Foods rich in lysine include many vegetables, legumes, turkey, chicken, fish, and potatoes.

ꙮ *Sugar products and alcohol* should be limited due to their immune-suppressive effects.

Nutritional supplements

ꙮ *L-Lysine* is an amino acid that may help prevent or reduce the severity of herpes outbreaks. Therapeutic dosage is 1,000 mg taken three times daily between meals *during outbreaks* and 1,000 to 1,500 mg daily as a preventive dosage.

ꙮ *Vitamin C* supports the immune system. A dosage of 2,000 mg and higher is therapeutic, while 1,000 to 2,000 mg can be used for prevention.

ꙮ *Zinc* supports the immune system to prevent infection and works to speed up healing of acute herpes infections. Therapeutic dosage is 50 mg daily, while 25 mg is a preventive dose.

ꙮ *Vitamin E* promotes tissue healing. Vitamin E oil can be applied topically to the lesions (when dry); 400 IU taken orally promotes healing.

ꙮ *Selenium* helps prevent virus replication. Take 200 to 400 mcg daily for prevention.

ꙮ *Propolis* is a bee product that proved, in one study, more effective than acyclovir in healing genital herpes lesions. Apply as a cream or spray three times daily.

Herbal

ꙮ *Lomatium* has an antiviral effect and can help reduce the length and severity of an acute herpes outbreak. Take 30 drops every two to three hours at the first sign of symptoms and use until lesions have healed.

ꙮ *Lemon Balm* can be used topically to speed up healing of herpes infection. Apply the cream three times daily to lesions during acute infections.

> ❧ **Licorice Root** has antiviral and immune-boosting properties. It can be taken internally at 30 drops or 250 mg three times daily, or applied as a topical gel.

NOTE: Higher doses of Licorice Root should not be used if you have high blood pressure.

Homeopathy

> ❧ **Rhus Toxicodendron** is for itchy, burning outbreaks. Take two pellets of 30C potency three times daily.

> ❧ **Herpes Nosode** is the homeopathic version of a vaccination against herpes outbreaks. Take a 30C-potency pellet twice daily for three days.

HYPOTHYROIDISM

It seems we have a silent epidemic among women. According to some holistic physicians, as many as one in two women has an underfunctioning thyroid that may not be picked up by blood tests. Classic symptoms of low thyroid function include low body temperature (consistently below 98.6 degrees F); fatigue; chills; dry, coarse skin; tendency to gain weight; tendency to be constipated; poor memory; and depression. However, joint pain, hair loss, brittle nails, menstrual irregularity, high cholesterol, weak heart, and other systemic problems can also result from an underactive thyroid.

The most common conventional cause of hypothyroidism is a condition known as Hashimoto thyroiditis, wherein the immune system attacks the thyroid gland. A high estrogen-to-progesterone ratio can also suppress the thyroid, so a hormonal imbalance is often behind the problem among women in menopause. This can result from lack of ovulation, sole use of estrogen for HRT (as is commonly done with Premarin®), or exposure to environmental pollutants, such as pesticides, that mimic the effects of estrogen. A deficiency of DHEA, a stress hormone, also weakens thyroid function over time. Finally, emotional stress can be a contributing factor to a sluggish thyroid.

Nutrition

ᴥ *Natural sources of iodine* (which is required for thyroid hormone synthesis) are recommended. Try sea vegetables such as wakame, agar, nori, kombu, kelp, and hijiki.

ᴥ *Avoid consuming large amounts of cabbage, Brussels sprouts, soy, and broccoli in their raw state,* as they can suppress thyroid function.

NOTE: You can eat these foods in liberal amounts if cooked or steamed, which inactivates the substances that cause problems with the thyroid.

Nutritional supplements

ᴥ *High-potency multivitamins* are important to coping with this problem, as many vitamins and minerals are needed to produce thyroid hormone, including vitamins A, E, C, all of the B's, selenium, and zinc.

ᴥ *L-tyrosine* is an amino acid used to manufacture thyroid hormone. Take 500 mg twice daily between meals. It is best used under the guidance of a nutritional doctor.

ᴥ *Essential fatty acids* are involved in the production of thyroid hormones. Take one to two tablespoons of flaxseed oil or a blended formula that also contains GLA.

ᴥ *Thyroid glandular* stimulates thyroid function. Use it by itself or in conjunction with pituitary glandular. Average dose is one or two tablets twice daily between meals.

Herbal

ᴥ *Kelp* is a natural source of iodine. It may be helpful in mild cases of hypothyroidism. Take 1,000 mg daily.

Homeopathy

ᴥ *Thyroid 3X* may be helpful. Take two pellets twice daily to stimulate thyroid function.

Hormonal

🍃 *Take your temperature* three times throughout a day. If it averages below 98.6 degrees F, you may have an underfunctioning thyroid.

🍃 *Natural thyroid hormone replacement* such as Armour Thyroid® or Thyrolar® is preferable to commonly used synthetic medication such as Synthroid®, which contains an incomplete form of thyroid hormone. Some women require T3 therapy (a time released form works best).

🍃 *Natural estrogen and progesterone* should replace synthetics, as Premarin® has been shown to suppress thyroid function.

🍃 *DHEA* supplementation can be used if testing shows levels are low.

Lifestyle

🍃 *Exercise* stimulates thyroid function.

INSOMNIA

Problems with sleep can begin or intensify with menopause. Some women have trouble falling asleep, while others wake up during the night or early morning and have trouble getting back to sleep. Hormones may be involved, as may other factors such as hypoglycemia, stress, and stimulating substances.

Conventional therapy relies on tranquilizing medications such as Valium® (diazepam). Antidepressants are also sometimes used. The obvious problems with these medications are side effects and addictiveness. Natural therapies avoid these problems.

Nutrition

🍃 *Avoid stimulating substances* such as caffeine and sugars in the evening.

🍃 *Alcohol* can impair REM (deep) sleep and should be avoided.

🍃 *A complex carbohydrate snack,* such as oatmeal, before bedtime may help you get to sleep.

෨ *Tryptophan* is a natural substance that helps make you drowsy enough for sleep. You'll find it in cheese and turkey.

Nutritional supplements

෨ *Calcium and magnesium* promote relaxation. Take 500 mg of each with the evening meal.

෨ *5HTP* is effective for insomnia. Take 100 to 200 mg a half hour before bedtime with some fruit juice.

NOTE: Iron-deficiency anemia can cause insomnia, but do not supplement with iron unless your bloodwork shows a deficiency.

Herbal

෨ *Chamomile tea* promotes relaxation. Drink a cup one hour before bedtime.

෨ *Passionflower or Valerian* (30 drops of either) can be helpful if taken a half hour before bedtime.

Hormonal

෨ *Estrogen and progesterone balance* is important in treating the underlying cause of insomnia with menopausal women. Menotype B's often respond well to natural progesterone.

෨ *Melatonin* promotes sleep. Typical dose is 0.5 mg a half hour before bedtime.

෨ *Acupuncture* can be helpful for chronic insomnia.

Lifestyle

෨ *Regular exercise, prayer, and other stress-reduction techniques* help promote sleep.

LOW LIBIDO

Low sex drive is frequently an issue among women experiencing menopause. It has been estimated that over 80 percent of postmenopausal women experience a decrease in libido. I find there are two main causes: physical factors and relationship/emotional factors.

A hormone imbalance can be at the root of such physical factors as vaginal dryness and painful sex (low levels of estrogen, progesterone, or testosterone can lead to thinning and drying of the vaginal walls). Physical factors tend to be more of a problem with menotype C and some B.

Relationship problems in a marriage or partnership can also greatly contribute to libido problems, but mental/emotional stress can also impair even libido, when your love relationship is a good one. Finally, a partner who's disinterested or unromantic can certainly dampen your interest in sex.

Nutrition

- ›◦ *Soy foods* may be helpful in improving vaginal lubrication. Tofu, miso, and tempeh should be included in the diet. Fermented soy protein powders may be helpful as well.

Nutritional supplements

- ›◦ *Vitamin E* may be helpful for menotypes A and B for mild vaginal dryness. Take 800 to 1,200 IU daily.

Herbal

- ›◦ *Black Cohosh* improves mild to moderate vaginal dryness. It is especially helpful for menotypes A and B. Recommended dosage is 80 to 160 mg daily of a 2.5% triterpene glycoside extract.

- ›◦ **Damiana** *(Turnera diffusa)* has been historically used by herbalists for low libido, although scientific research is lacking. Dosage is 500 mg three times daily.

Homeopathy

- ›◦ *Sepia* is the most common remedy for low sex drive (see Chapter 7 for a further description). Take two pellets of 30C potency twice daily for one week. If you show improvement, use as needed.

Hormonal

- ≈ *Natural progesterone and/or DHEA* may help menotype B improve libido if levels are low.

- ≈ *Natural hormone replacement* may give menotype C relief.

- ≈ *Estriol or testosterone cream* as prescribed by your doctor can help some women.

PMS

Premenstrual syndrome generally occurs during the last 14 days of a woman's menstrual cycle. The symptoms vary from woman to woman. Common ones include anxiety, irritability, mood swings, crying spells, and depression. In addition, physical symptoms including bloating, breast tenderness, headaches, fatigue, and sweet cravings appear or intensify during this time of the month. Relief comes with the menstrual flow.

Many theories attempt to explain the causes of PMS, including neurotransmitter imbalance (serotonin decrease after ovulation) and hormone imbalance (high estrogen relative to progesterone, and increased prolactin levels).

Conventional therapy offers the birth-control pill, antidepressant and anti-anxiety medications, and synthetic progesterone for relief. However, not only do natural therapies alleviate symptoms, but they treat underlying causes as well. Keep in mind that it can take two cycles for noticeable improvement to occur.

Nutrition

- ≈ *A high-fiber diet* helps to expel excess levels of estrogen that may be a factor in PMS.

- ≈ *Fermented soy foods* are recommended for their hormone-balancing properties. Foods that improve liver function, such as beets, carrots, dandelion greens, and cruciferous vegetables, help the liver metabolize hormones more effectively.

❧ *Sugar products* should be avoided, especially during the last two weeks of the cycle.

❧ *Caffeine and alcohol* should be limited as they deplete the body of B6, magnesium, and calcium, all of which are important in preventing PMS.

❧ *Salt* intake should be restricted among women who experience water retention.

Nutritional supplements

❧ *Magnesium* has proven in several studies to help prevent PMS by assisting the liver in estrogen metabolism. Recommended dosage is 500 mg daily.

❧ *Calcium* can also help relieve PMS. Recommended dosage is 1,000 mg daily.

❧ *Vitamin B6* is excellent for treating PMS because it helps the liver metabolize hormones and is involved in the synthesis of serotonin. Recommended dosage is 50 to 100 mg daily.

❧ *GLA* is an essential fatty acid that has proven effective in preventing PMS. Take 200 mg of GLA daily as part of an essential fatty acid complex that also contains omega-3 fatty acids.

❧ *Vitamin E* helps with estrogen metabolism and works well for breast tenderness. Take 800 to 1,200 IU daily.

❧ *Indole-3 carbinole* assists the liver in detoxifying the blood of estrogen and other hormones. Take 300 mg daily.

❧ *D-glucarate* also assists the liver in breaking down hormones, such as estrogen. Take 500 to 1,500 mg daily.

Herbal

❧ *Vitex (Chasteberry)* can help balance estrogen and progesterone ratios. Several studies confirm its effectiveness for PMS. Take a daily dosage of 40 to 80 drops of a standardized tincture, or 240 mg of a 0.6% aucubin standardized capsule extract.

NOTE: Do not use Vitex (Chasteberry) along with birth-control pills.

- *Milk Thistle* promotes liver detoxification. Take 200 mg of a 85% silymarin extract three times daily.

- *Dandelion Leaf* can be used to relieve water retention. Take 300 mg or 30 drops three times daily on the days when you feel swollen or bloated.

- *Passionflower* helps reduce anxiety and irritability. Take 300 to 500 mg or 30 drops three times daily for acute bouts of these symptoms.

- *Dong Quai* is helpful for relieving breast tenderness and cramping. Take 30 to 500 mg twice daily the last seven days of your cycle.

Hormonal

- *Natural progesterone cream* alleviates PMS. I recommend it when other natural therapies are not working. Apply one-quarter teaspoon twice daily beginning after ovulation (day 15) until one day before your period begins.

UTERINE FIBROIDS

Approximately 50 percent of all women experience benign uterine fibroids, which are overgrowths of the smooth muscle and connective tissue inside the uterus. These growths are the most common reason why women undergo major surgery.

Estrogen stimulation probably causes them. They tend to increase in size during perimenopause (when progesterone levels are getting lower) and shrink postmenopausally (when there is less estrogen stimulation). They can also grow during pregnancy.

Most fibroids do not cause any symptoms. However, they can cause abnormal uterine bleeding, a feeling of pressure and heaviness, painful sex, increased urinary frequency, backache, and enlargement of the abdomen.

Conventional therapy uses the birth-control pill, Lupron® (a drug that suppresses ovarian production of estrogen), and surgery.

Natural medicine can be helpful in reducing symptoms (such as heavy bleeding) until a woman is postmenopausal, at which time fibroids generally shrink on their own. In some cases, natural treatments can shrink fibroids but not always. Hormone balancing is the key to successful treatment. Surgery may be required for larger fibroids, or when heavy bleeding and other symptoms cannot be brought under control.

Nutrition

- *A high-fiber diet* helps to expel excess levels of estrogen that are implicated in fibroids.

- *Fermented soy foods* are recommended for their hormone-balancing properties.

- *Foods that improve liver function* such as beets, carrots, dandelion greens, and cruciferous vegetables help the liver metabolize hormones more effectively.

Nutritional supplements

- *Vitamin E* helps with estrogen metabolism and works well for breast tenderness. Take 800 to 1,200 IU daily.

- *Indole-3 carbinole* assists in the liver's detoxification of estrogen and other hormones. Take 300 mg daily.

- *D-glucarate* assists in the liver's breakdown of hormones, such as estrogen. Take 500 to 1,500 mg daily.

NOTE: Iron may be required if there has been heavy or prolonged bleeding.

Herbal

- *Vitex (Chasteberry)* can help balance estrogen and progesterone ratios. Take a daily dosage of 40 to 80 drops of a standardized tincture, or 240 mg of a 0.6% aucubin standardized capsule extract.

NOTE: Do not use Vitex (Chasteberry) along with birth-control pills.

Homeopathy

ਊ *Fraxinus americanus* may help. Take two pellets of a 6X, 12X, or 6C potency three times daily for at least eight weeks.

Hormonal

ਊ *Natural progesterone cream* can be beneficial. Apply one-quarter teaspoon twice daily three weeks on and one week off. If you have regular periods, then do not apply the cream for the week you have your period.

VAGINITIS

Approximately 10 percent of visits by women to their doctor are for vaginitis. This refers to either an infection or irritation of the vaginal tissues. In postmenopausal women, atrophic vaginitis can occur where vaginal dryness leads to increased problems with irritation and infection. Atrophic vaginitis occurs among menotype C's and to a lesser degree, menotype B's. Systemic or local hormone therapy is effective.

Infectious vaginitis is usually due to bacterial vaginosis, trichomoniasis, or candidiasis. This section will focus on the common problem of candidiasis, also referred to as yeast infection. Vaginal yeast infections are characterized by itching and a cheese- or cream-like discharge. Vaginal soreness and irritation are common.

Conventional treatment offers anti-yeast vaginal or oral medications.

Natural medicine focuses on eradicating the infection and simultaneously normalizing the vaginal environment so that reinfection is less likely.

Nutrition

ਊ *Sugar products and alcohol products* should be avoided. For some women, sensitivities to foods, such as dairy products, can be a problem.

&. *Cultured yogurt* can help if dairy products are not a problem, as it promotes the growth of friendly bacteria that keep down yeast populations.

&. *Garlic and onions* can be eaten liberally for their anti-yeast properties.

Nutritional supplements

&. *Boric acid powder* capsules destroy *Candida* (yeast). Insert a capsule intravaginally morning and evening for four to six days.

&. *Vitamin E gel* can be applied to the external genitalia to prevent burning. If the problem is chronic, use one to two times daily for two to three weeks.

&. *Lactobacillus acidophilus* is a good bacterium that fights yeast. Take orally at 6 to 8 billion organisms per day (listed on container) and insert a capsule intravaginally before bedtime for four to eight days.

&. *Vitamin C* at a dose of 1,000 mg two to three times daily will give your immune system support.

Herbal

&. *Echinacea* stimulates the immune system and has proven effective against yeast. Take 30 to 60 drops, or 1,000 mg three times daily for seven days.

Homeopathy

&. *Kreosotum* is for vaginal yeast infections where there is unbearable itching. Take two pellets of 30C potency twice daily for five days.

Hormonal

&. *Black Cohosh and Vitex* can be helpful in reestablishing hormonal balance, which plays an important role in the susceptibility to vaginal yeast infections.

• *Natural progesterone,* when used the week before the menses, can also help restore hormone balance. I have seen the birth-control pill and Premarin® increase some women's susceptibility to this problem.

$\mathcal{R}$ESOURCES

FURTHER INFORMATION

Angela Stengler, N.D., and Mark Stengler, N.D., can be contacted for any of the following:

- To order saliva hormone analysis or nutritional test kits that can be done in the comfort of your home.
- For clinic or phone consultation.
- To request for speaking engagement or media interview.

The Stenglers can be reached at:

La Jolla Whole Health Medical Clinic
8950 Villa La Jolla Drive, Suite 1172
La Jolla, CA 92037
(858) 450-7120
www.thenaturalphysician.com

SALIVA AND HAIR TESTING LABS

Great Smokies Diagnostic Laboratory
63 Zillicoa Street
Asheville, NC 28801-1072
(800) 522-4762
www.gsdl.com

Diagnos Techs
6620 S. 192nd Place, Bldg. J
Kent, WA 98032
(800) 878-3787
www.diagnostechs.com

Aeron LifeCycles Laboratory
1933 Davis Street, Suite 310
San Leandro, CA 94577
(800) 631-7900
www.aeron.com

URINALYSIS LAB

Urine Hormone Testing
Meridian Valley Laboratory
515 West Harrison Street, Suite 9
Kent, WA 98032
(253) 859-8700

COMPOUNDING PHARMACISTS

Professional Compounding Centers of America
9901 S. Wilcrest
Houston, TX 77099
(800) 331-2498
Fax: (281) 495-0602
www.pccarx.com

International Academy of Compounding Pharmacists (IACP)
P.O. Box 1365
Sugar Land, TX 77487
(800) 927-4227
Fax: (281) 495-0602
www.iacprx.org

NATUROPATHIC DOCTORS

American Association of Naturopathic Physicians
8201 Greensboro Drive, Suite 300
McLean, VA 22102
(877) 969-2267
www.naturopathic.org

American Association for the Advancement of Medicine
P.O. Box 3427
Laguna Hills, CA 92654
(800) 532-3688

HOMEOPATHIC REFERRAL AGENCIES

National Center for Homeopathy
801 North Fairfax Street, Suite 306
Alexandria, VA 22314
(703) 548-7790
www.homeopathic.org

Homeopathic Academy of Naturopathic Physicians
12132 Southeast Foster Place
Portland, OR 97266
(503) 761-3298

RECOMMENDED READING

Natural Hormone Replacement: For Women over 45 by Jonathan Wright, M.D. and John Morgenthaler (Petaluma, CA: Smart Publications, 1997).

The Natural Physician's Healing Therapies by Mark Stengler, N.D. (Paramus, NJ: Prentice Hall Press, 2001).

Natural Woman, Natural Menopause by Marcus Laux, N.D. and Christine Conrad (New York: HarperCollins, 1997).

What Your Doctor May Not Tell You About Premenopause by John R. Lee, M.D., Jesse Hanley, M.D., and Virginia L. Hopkins (New York: Warner Books, 1999).

Women's Encyclopedia of Natural Medicine by Tori Hudson, N.D. (Lincolnwood, IL: Keats/NTC/Contemporary Publishing Group, Inc., 1999).

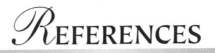EFERENCES

INTRODUCTION

Page xv . . . "A study published in *The Journal* of the American Medical Association . . ." Schairer C., PhD; Lubin J, PhD; Troisi R., ScD; Sturgeon S., DrPH; Brinton L., PhD; Hoover R., MD. Menopausal estrogen and estrogen-progestin replacement therapy and breast cancer risk. *JAMA* 2000; 283:485–491.

Page xvi . . . "The 1998 HERS (Heart and Estrogen/Progestin Replacement Study) study looked at over 2700 postmenopausal women with coronary artery disease and found that taking hormones did not reduce their risk of death." Hulley S, Grady D, Bush T et al. Randomized trial of estrogen plus progestin for secondary prevention of coronary heart disease in postmenopausal women. *JAMA* 1998;280:605–613.

Page xvi... "It should come as no surprise that the American Heart Association recently issued a report..." Mossa L et al. Hormone Replacement Therapy and Cardiovascular Disease. *Circulation* 2001;104:499–503.

CHAPTER 1

Page 7 . . . "In fact, one study found that rural Mayan Indians going through mejopause showed none of the symptoms we typically associate with it." Martin MC, et al. Menopause without symptoms: The endocrinology of menopause among rural Mayan Indians. *Am J Obstet Gynecol* 1993;168:1839–1845.

Page 9 . . . "The three most common reasons for hysterectomy are uterine fibroids, endometriosis, and uterine prolapse." CDC website. August 08, 1997/46(SS-4);1–15 Hysterectomy Surveillance—United States. 1980–1993.

CHAPTER 3

Page 61 . . . "There is some literature that supports the idea that the hormone LH (lutenizing hormone) is lowered with black cohosh supplementation." Duker EM et al. Effects of extracts from Cimicifuga racemosa on gonadotropin release in menopausal women and ovariectomized rats. *Planta Medica* 1991;57:420–424.

Page 61 . . . "A study by Stolze involved 131 doctors and 629 female patients." Stolze H. An alternative to treat menopausal complaints. *Gyne* 1982;3:4–16.

Page 61 . . . "In another study, 80 menopausal women were given either black cohosh synthetic estrogen, or placebo for 12 weeks." Stoll W. Phytopharmacon influences atrophic vaginal epithelium: Double-blind study—Cimicifuga vs. estrogenic substances. *Therapeutikon* 1987;1:23–30.

Page 63 . . . "Researchers have also studied women who were making a transition from hormones to black cohosh." Petho A. Menopausal complaints: Changeover of a hormone treatment to a herbal gynecological remedy practicable? *Arzliche Praxis* 1987;38(47):1551–1553.

Page 63 . . . "Clinical studies involving more than 1,700 patients over a three- to six-month period showed excellent tolerance of black cohosh. Harnischfeger G, Stolze H. Black cohosh. *Notabene Medici* 10:446–450, 1980.

Page 63 . . . "One study showed that breast cancer cells whose growth is dependent on estrogen are not stimulated by black cohosh." Examination of the proliferative potential of phytopharmaceuticals with estrogen-mimicking acting in breast carcinoma. *Arch Gynecol Obstet* 1993;254:817–818.

Page 64 . . . "Vitex may raise progesterone levels." Anmann W. Removing an obstipation using Agnolyt. *Ther Gegenw* 1965;104:1263–1265.

Page 65 . . . "Well-known herbalist Christopher Hobbs comments in his book *Vitex: The Women's Herb,* 'Vitex and preparations containing the herb are the most widely-used natural medicine in Europe for helping to relieve unpleasant symptoms that may occur before, during, and after menopause, being recommended by herbalists and physicians alike.' Hobbs C. *Vitex: The Women's Herb.* Santa Cruz: Botanica Press, 1996, p. 14.

Page 65 . . . "It does contain a steroidal saponin known as diosgenin. Diosgenin acts as the precursor for the pharmaceutical synthesis of estrogen, progesterone, and pregnenolone." Felter HW. The eclectic *Materia Medica. Pharmacology and Therapeutics* 1922; 344; and Mowrey D. *The Scientific Validation of Herbal Medicine.* New Canaan, CT: Keats Publishing, Inc., 1986; pp. 107–115, 151–156.

Page 65 . . . "It has also been shown to mildly lower triglycerides (fats) and raise HDL ("good") cholesterol in the blood." Araghinikam M et al. Antioxidant activity of dioscorea and dehydroepiandrosterone (DHEA) in older humans. *Life Sci* 1996;11:147–157.

Page 67 . . . "Licorice contains isoflavones that have estrogen and progesterone balancing compounds." Kumigai A et al. Effect of glycyrrhizin on estrogen action. *Endocrinologia Japnica* 1967;14(1):34–38.

Page 68 . . . "According to herbalist Rosemary Gladstar, 'Hops contain high concentrations of plant hormones that have estrogen-like effects on the female system.'" Gladstar R. *Herbal Healing for Women*. New York: Fireside Books, 1993, p. 258.

Page 70 . . . "Rehmannia is used in Chinese herbal medicine for conditions such as irregular menses, palpitations, insomnia, dizziness, night sweats, vaginal dryness, and hot flashes." Revised by Gamble A and Kaptchuk TJ. *Chinese Herbal Medicine: Materia Medica*. Seattle, WA: Eastland Press, 1993, p.328.

Page 71 . . . "A study by Nestel et al examined the effects of an isoflavone extract from red clover on the elasticity of the large arteries, which typically declines after menopause." Nestel PJ et al. Isoflavones from red clover improve systemic arterial compliance but not plasma lipids in menopausal women. *J Clin Endocrinol Metab* March 1999;84(3):895–898.

Page 72 . . . "In a 12-week study of 111 menopausal women, by Grube et al, nearly 80 percent reported improved psychological symptoms after treatment with St. John's Wort extract." Grube B, Walper A, Wheatley D. St. John's Wort extract: Efficacy for menopausal symptoms of psychological origin. *Adv Ther* Jul–Aug 1999;16(4):177–186.

Page 73 . . . "In a clinical trial by Vorbach et al, 209 patients with severe depression were given either St. John's Wort or the antidepressant drug imipramine." Vorbach EU et al. Efficacy and tolerability of St. John's Wort extract L1 160 versus imipramine in patients with severe depressive episodes according to ICD-10. *Pharmacopsychiatry* 1997;30(Suppl):81–85.

Page 73 . . . "In a double-blind, placebo-controlled study by Warnecke . . ." Warnecke G. Psychosomatic dysfunctions in the female climacteric. Clinical effectiveness and tolerance of Kava extract US 1490. *Fortschr med* Feb10; 109(4):119–122.

Page 76 . . . "A double-blind, cross-over study on university students in Italy, by D'Angelo et al, compared Panax ginseng to a placebo." D'Angelo L et al. A double-blind, placebo controlled clinical study on the effect of a standardized ginseng extract on psychomotor performance in healthy volunteers. *J Ethnopharmacol* 1986;16:15–22.

Page 77 . . . "A 1998 study in *The New England Journal of Medicine* demonstrated that cranberry prevents the fimbriae (analogous to arms and hands of bacteria) from attaching to the urinary tract walls." Howell AB, Vorsa N, Marderosian AD et al. Inhibition of the adherence of P-fimbriated *Escerichia coli* to uroepithelial-cell surfaces by proanthocyanadin extracts from cranberries. *New Engl J Med* 1998;339(15):1085–1086.

Page 77 . . . "A study by Wilson et al. examined the effects of cranberry extract on low-density lipoproteins (LDL) oxidation." Wilson T et al. Cranberry extract inhibits low density lipoprotein oxidation. *Life Sci* 1998; 62(24):PL381–PL386.

CHAPTER 4

Page 81 . . . "Environmental toxins are suspect as are the effect of stress, and anxiety can lower stimulation of the thyroid by the pituitary gland." *Textbook of Medical Physiology,* 8th Edition. Philadelphia: W.B. Saunders Company, 1991, p. 837.

Page 87 . . . "According to the *Physician's Desk Reference,* Premarin® 'contains estrone, equilin, and 17-dihydroequilin, together with smaller amounts of 17-estradiol, equilenin, and 17-dihydroequilenin.' *Physician's Desk Reference,* 52nd Edition. Montvale, NJ: Medical Economics Company, 1998, p. 311.

Page 87 . . . "According to one published study, equilin and equilenin make up approximately 20% of Premarin®, quite a substantial amount." Zhang F, Bolton JL. Synthesis of the equine estrogen metabolites 2-hydroxyequilin and 2-hydroxyequilenin. *Chem Res Toxicol* Feb 1999;12(2):200–203.

Page 87 . . . "Several *in vitro* studies have shown that Premarin® metabolites damage cell DNA and according to researchers may have carcinogenic effects." Pisha E, Lui X, Constantinou AI, Bolton JL. Evidence that a metabolite of equine estrogens, 4-hydroxyequilenin, induces cellular transformation in vitro. *Chem Res Toxicol* Jan 2001;14(1):82–90. Zhang F, Chen Y, Pisha E,

Shen L, Xiong Y, van Breemen RB, Bolton JL. The major metabolite of equilin, 4-hydroxyequilin, autoxidizes to an o-quinone which isomerizes to the potent cytotoxin 4-hydroxyequilenin-o-quinone. *Chem Res Toxicol* Feb 1999;12(2):204–213. Zhang F, Bolton JL. Synthesis of the equine estrogen metabolites 2-hydroxyequilin and 2-hydroxyequilenin. *Chem Res Toxicol* Feb 1999;12(2):200–203. Chen Y, Liu X, Pisha E, Constantinou AI, Hua Y, Shen L, van Breemen RB, Elguindi EC, Blond SY, Zhang F, Bolton JL. A metabolite of equine estrogens, 4-hydroxyequilenin, induces DNA damage and apoptosis in breast cancer cell lines. *Chem Res Toxicol* May 2000; 13(5):342–350.

Page 90 . . . "However, a study of postmenopausal women who were current or recent users of the combination of synthetic estrogen and synthetic progesterone had a relatively higher risk of breast cancer than women who take only estrogen." Schairer C, PhD; Lubin J, PhD; Troisi R, ScD; Sturgeon S, DrPH; Brinton L, PhD; Hoover R, MD. Menopausal estrogen and estrogen-progestin replacement therapy and breast cancer risk. *JAMA* 2000; 283:485–449.

Page 90 . . . "Side effects associated with synthetic progesterone products such as Provera® include blood clots, fluid retention, breast tenderness, acne, hair loss, and hirsuitism, breakthrough bleeding, nausea, jaundice, depression, edema, weight change, and anaphylaxis. Studies on beagle dogs with medroxyprogesterone acetate showed that some developed breast nodules, some of which were cancerous." *Physician's Desk Reference,* 52nd Edition. Montvale, NJ: Medical Economics Company, 1998, p. 822.

Page 91 . . . "The Nurses' Health Study which involved close to 122,000 women found that women who took only estrogen had a 36% increase in breast cancer risk, those on the combination of estrogen and progestin had a 50% increased risk, and those on progestin alone had a 240% increase." Colditz G, Hankinson S, Hunter D et al. The use of estrogens and progestins and the risk of breast cancer in postmenopausal women. *New Engl J Med* 1995; 332:1589–1593.

Page 92 . . . "A study completed by St. Luke's Hospital in Bethlemen, PA, found that using progesterone cream prevented build up of the endometrium among postmenopausal women who were taking synthetic estrogen (Premarin®)." Anasti JN, Leonetti HB, Wilson KJ. Topical progesterone cream has antiproliferative effect on estrogen-stimulated endometrium. *Obstet Gynecol* Apr 2001; 1997(4 Suppl 1):S10.

CHAPTER 5

Page 105 . . . "Following are some foods and their fiber content." Marlett J, Cheung T. Database and quick methods of assessing typical dietary fiber intakes using data for 228 commonly consumed foods. *J Am Diet Assoc* 1997;97:1139–1147.

Page 107 . . . "Research has shown that the average American consumes 125 pounds of sugar a year." Sanchex A et al. Role of sugars in human neutrophilic phagocytosis. *Am J Clinical Nutrition* 1973; 26:1180–1184.

Page 111 . . . "One 12-week study of postmenopausal women..." Albertazzi P, Pansini F, Bonaccorsi G, Zanotti L, Forini E, De Aloysio D. The effect of dietary soy supplementation on hot flushes. *Obstet Gynecol* Jan 1998; 91(1):6–11.

Page 114 . . . "We know that 75% of adults have some degree of lactase deficiency, except those who are of northwest European descent for whom the incidence is less than 20%." *The Merck Manual,* 17th Edition, 1999, p. 298.

CHAPTER 6

Page 124 . . . "The Nurses' Health Study involved 87,000 women and found those who took vitamin E for two years or more had a 41-percent reduction in the risk of heart disease." Stampfer MJ et al. Vitamin E consumption and the risk of coronary artery disease in women. *New Engl J Med* 1993;328:1444–1448.

Page 125 . . . "A recent study reported in the *Lancet* medical journal found a small increase in vitamin C intake could produce a substantial reduction in cardiovascular mortality." Riemersma MA et al. Plasma ascorbic acid and risk of heart disease and cancer. *Lancet* 2001;357:657–663.

CHAPTER 7

Page 134 . . . "According to Dana Ullman, co-author of *Everybody's Guide to Homeopathic Medicines,* over 70,000 registered homeopaths practice in India. . . . In France, more than 6,000 physicians practice homeopathy and over 18,000 pharmacies sell homeopathic remedies." Cummings S, Ullman D. *Everybody's Guide to Homeopathic Medicines.* Los Angeles: Jeremy P. Tarcher, Inc., 1984.

CHAPTER 8

Page 142 . . . "One Swedish study of almost 800 women found that only 5% of highly physically active women experienced severe hot flashes as compared with 14–16% of women who had little or no weekly exercise." Ivarsson T, Spetz AC, Hammar M. Physical exercise and vasomotor symptoms in postmenopausal women. *Maturitas* Jun 3, 1998;29(2):139–146.

Page 142 . . . "The Nurses' Health Study, which involved 72,488 female nurses . . ." Hu FB, Stampfer MJ, Colditz GA, Ascherio A, Rexrode KM, Willett WC, Manson JE. Physical activity and risk of stroke in women. *JAMA* Jun 14, 2000; 283(22):2961–2967.

Page 142 . . . "Two studies by Australian scientists looked at the impact of exercise on menopausal symptoms." Slaven L, Lee C. Mood and symptom reporting among middle-aged women: The relationship between menopausal status, hormone replacement therapy, and exercise participation. *Health Psychol* May 1997; 16(3):203–298.

Page 144 . . . "One study investigated the effect of exercise on adults with low back pain." Moffett JK, Torgerson D, Bell-Syer S, Jackson D, Llewlyn-Phillips H, Farrin A, Barber J. Randomised controlled trial of exercise for low back pain: Clinical outcomes, costs, and preferences. *BMJ* Jul 31, 1999; 319(7205):279–283.

Page 144 . . . "One study followed 132 people between the ages of 24 and 76."Van Boxtel MP, Paas FG, Houx PJ, Adam JJ, Teeken JC, Jolles J. Aerobic capacity and cognitive performance in a cross-sectional aging study. *Med Sci Sports Exerc* Oct 1997; 29(10):1357–1365.

Page 154 . . . "One study focused on 40,417 postmenopausal Iowa women..." Kushi LH et al. Physical activity and mortality in post-menopausal women. *JAMA* 1997; 277:1287–1292.

Page 155 . . . "One review looked at several studies on strength training in older people." Hurley BF, Roth SM. Strength training in the elderly: Effects on risk factors for age-related diseases. *Sports Med* Oct 2000; 30(4):249–268.

Page 155 . . . "Consider a University of Alabama at Birmingham study on older women and weight lifting." Hunter GR, Treuth MS, Weinsier RI, Kekes-Szabo T, Kell SH, Roth DL, Nicholson C. The effects of strength training on older women's ability to perform daily tasks. *J Am Geriatr Soc* Jul 1995; 43(7):756–760.

CHAPTER 10

Page 177 . . . "Following are some women-specific statistics about heart disease from the American Heart Association." American Heart Association website, 2001. www.americanheart.org.

Page 178 . . . "The authors of this study concluded, 'Among women, adherence to lifestyle guidelines involving diet, exercise, and abstinence from smoking is associated with a very low risk of coronary heart disease.'" Stampfer MJ, Hu FB, Manson JE, Rimm EB, Willett WC. Primary prevention of coronary heart disease in women through diet and lifestyle. *N Engl J Med* Jul 6, 2000;343(1):16–22.

Page 179 . . . "The Framingham study found that people with cholesterol levels below 175 mg/dl had less than half the rate of heart attack as compared to those whose levels were 250 to 275 mg/dl." Anderson KM, Castelli WP, Levy D. Cholesterol and mortality. 30 years of follow-up from the Framingham study. *JAMA* Apr 24, 1987;257(16):2176–2180.

Page 180 . . . "A review of 16 studies (952 people) found that garlic lowered total cholesterol levels by 12 percent after one to three months of treatment." Silagy C, Neil A. Garlic as a lipid-lowering agent—A meta-analysis. *J Royal Coll Physicians* 1994;28(1):39–45.

Page 182 . . . "One study of almost 28,000 showed that only 86 persons reported adverse effects, of which the most frequent complaint was weight loss." Fernandez L et al. Policosanol: Results of a postmarketing surveillance study of 27,879 patients. *Curr Ther Res* 1998; 59:7717–7722.

Page 182 . . . "Several studies have shown elevated Lp(a) to be one of the best predictors of coronary artery disease." Merz B. Is it time to include lipoprotein analysis in cholesterol screening. Medical news and perspectives. *JAMA* 1989;261(4):496–497. Hearn JA, DeMaio SJ et al. Predictive value of lipoprotein(a) and other serum lipoproteins in the angiographic diagnosis of coronary artery disease. *Am J Cardiol* 1990; 66(17):1176–1180.

Page 183 . . . "Studies on women have shown it to be an independent risk factor for heart attacks." Knekt P, Alfthan G, Aromaa A, Heliovaara M,

Marniemi J, Rissanen H, Reunanen A. Homocysteine and major coronary events: A prospective population study amongst women. *J Intern Med* May 2001;249(5):461–465.

Page 184 . . . "The Women's Health Study found that hs-CRP was 'the single strongest predictor of risk' in women. It proved an even better predictor than LDL cholesterol." Ridker PM, Buring JE, Shih J, Matias M, Hennekens CH. Prospective study of C-reactive protein and the risk of future cardiovascular events among apparently healthy women. *Circulation* Aug 25, 1998;98(8):731–733.

Page 184 . . . "One study found that postmenopausal hormone replacement increased the levels of C-reactive protein two times higher on average than women not on hormone replacement." Ridker PM, MD; Hennekens CH, MD; Rifai N, PhD; Buring JE, ScD; Manson JE, MD. Hormone replacement therapy and increased plasma concentration of C-reactive protein. *Circulation* August 17 1999;100:713–716.

Page 185 . . . "The Framingham Offspring Study measured fibrinogen in over 2,600 adults with an average age of about 55 years old. Similar results were found as in previous studies, which showed high fibrinogen levels are associated with a sixfold greater risk of developing coronary disease when combined with high LDL cholesterol, and a threefold greater independent risk of suffering a coronary event in patients with angina." Stec JJ, Silbershatz H, Tofler GH, Matheney TH, Sutherland P, Lipinska I, Massaro JM, Wilson PFW, Muller JE, D'Agostino RBD. Association of fibrinogen with cardiovascular risk factors and cardiovascular disease in the Framingham offspring population. *Circulation* 2000;102:1634–1638.

Page 188 . . . "Researchers at the University of Calgary evaluated metabolic and cardiovascular risk parameters in 57 women with PCOS. They found that 75 percent of the women with PCOS were hyperinsulinemic, and that 'cardiovascular risk factors [were] up to five times as prevalent' in the hyperinsulinemic group as in the PCOS patients with normal insulin levels." Mather KJ, Kwan F, Corenblum B. Hyperinsulinemia in polycystic ovary syndrome correlates with increased cardiovascular risk independent of obesity. *Fertil Steril* 2000;73(1):150–156.

Page 188 . . . "The Nurses' Health Study found that women with high blood pressure between the ages of 35 and 65 have a risk of coronary artery disease three and a half times women with normal blood pressure." Manson JE et al. A prospective study of obesity and risk of coronary heart disease in women. *N Engl J Med* 1990; 332(13):882–889.

Page 190 . . . "Researchers from the University of Maryland School of Medicine have found that laughter and a good sense of humor may actually provide some degree of protection against heart disease." Clark A, Seidler A, Miller M. Coronary disease and reduced situational humor-response: Is laughter cardioprotective? [Abstract] Presented at the 73rd Scientific Session of the American Heart Association, November 15, 2000, New Orleans.

Page 190 . . . "Studies have shown that people who suffer from depression have a greatly increased risk for heart disease. Depression has been shown to be a major determinant of cardiac death in those with or without symptomatic heart disease." Penninx BW, Beekman AT, Honig A, Deeg DJ, Schoevers RA, van Eijk JT, van Tilburg W. Depression and cardiac mortality: Results from a community-based longitudinal study. *Arch Gen Psychiatry* Mar 2001; 58(3):229–230).

Page 191 . . . "One large study found that at least one hour of walking per week predicted lower risk of heart disease. This was true for women at high risk for heart disease, including those who were overweight, had increased cholesterol levels, or were smokers." Lee IM, Rexrode KM, Cook NR, Manson JE, Buring JE. Physical activity and coronary heart disease in women: Is "no pain, no gain" passe? *JAMA* Mar 21, 2001; 285(11):1447–1454.

Page 192 . . . "Dr. Tori Hudson, a highly respected expert in women's health, poignantly states in her book *Women's Encyclopedia of Natural Medicine* the following, 'If one looks at the CAD (coronary artery disease) death rate for women, from birth to age 90, one finds it steadily increasing.'" Hudson T. *Women's Encyclopedia of Natural Medicine*. Lincolnwood, IL: Keats/NTC/Contemporary Publishing Group, Inc., 1999, pp. 106–107.

Page 193 . . . "It is well documented that estrogen replacement has benefits on many risk markers of cardiovascular disease. . . ." Wood MJ, Cox JL. HRT to prevent cardiovascular disease: What studies show, how to advise patients. *Postgrad Med* 2000:108(3):59–72.

Page 194 . . . "However, a commentary the medical journal *Postgraduate Medicine,* warns 'These observational data must be interpreted with caution. Patients who take estrogen may be more likely than other women to exercise, eat a low-fat diet, and live a healthy lifestyle. These factors are difficult to account for in observational studies.'" Wood MJ, Cox JL. HRT to prevent cardiovascular disease: What studies show, how to advise patients. *Postgrad Med* 2000;108(3):59–72.

Page 194 . . . "It is generally agreed upon that women who use estrogen tend to be leaner, be of higher socioeconomic status, have better access to healthcare, and visit their doctor more frequently." Hudson T. *Women's Encyclopedia of Natural Medicine.* Lincolnwood, IL: Keats/NTC/Contemporary Publishing Group, Inc., 1999, pp. 106.

Page 195 . . . "Dr. Dean Ornish has shown in studies that a vegetarian diet along with aerobic exercise, stress-management training, smoking cessation, and group psychosocial support, can reverse coronary artery disease." Ornish D et al. Intensive lifestyle changes for reversal of coronary heart disease. *JAMA* Dec 16, 1998;280(23):2001–2007.

Page 195 . . . "The Mediterranean diet (abundant in plant foods... and nuts, as well as olive oil, moderate amounts of fish, poultry, meat, dairy, eggs, and wine) has been shown to reduce the risk of a heart attack by as much as 70%." De Longeril M et al. *Circulation* 1999;99:779–785.

CHAPTER 11

Page 200 . . . "A recent survey of over 200 women aged 75 years and older revealed that 80% would rather be dead than experience the loss of independence and quality of life resulting from a bad hip fracture and subsequent admission to a nursing home." Salkeld G, Cameron ID, Cumming RG, Easter S, Seymour J, Kurrle SE, Quine S. Quality of life related to fear of falling and hip fracture in older women: A time trade off study. *BMJ* 2000;320:241–246.

Page 205 . . . "Fosamax® (Alendronate) is a non-hormonal drug that has been shown to increase bone density." *Physician's Desk Reference,* 52nd Edition. Montvale, NJ: Medical Economics Company, p. 1660.

Page 206 . . . "Calcitonin (Micalcin) is a hormone that works to stimulate bone formation and is used pharmaceutically as an injection, and more commonly as a nasal spray." *Physician's Desk Reference,* 52nd Edition. Montvale, NJ: Medical Economics Company, 1998, pp. 1660, 1881.

Page 208 . . . "A study of senior women (average age 79.5 years) looked at the effect of essential fatty acids on bone density." Kruger MC, Coetzer H, de Winter R, Gericke G, van Papendorp DH. Calcium, gamma-linolenic acid and eicosapentaenoic acid supplementation in senile osteoporosis. *Aging (Milano)* Oct 1998;10(5):385–394.

Page 208 . . . "One recent *in vitro* study showed that soy extract encouraged bone formation by stimulating bone-building osteoblasts." Choi EM, Suh KS, Kim YS, Choue RW, Koo SJ. Soybean ethanol extract increases the function of osteoblastic MC3T3-E1 cells. *Phytochemistry* Apr 2001;56(7):733–739.

Page 208 . . . "Another recent study on perimenopausal women demonstrated that soy halts bone loss in the lumbar spine." Alekel DL, Germain AS, Peterson CT, Hanson KB, Stewart JW, Toda T. Isoflavone-rich soy protein isolate attenuates bone loss in the lumbar spine of perimenopausal women. *Am J Clin Nutr* Sep 2000;72(3):679–680.

Page 209 . . . "A study in *The New England Journal of Medicine* that postmenopausal women who supplemented 1,000 mg of calcium daily experienced a 43-percent reduction in bone loss compared with women who weren't taking a calcium supplement." Reid IR et al. Effects of calcium supplementation on bone loss in postmenopausal women. *New Engl J Med* 1993;12:S11–16.

Page 211 . . . "One study looked at 249 healthy postmenopausal women with an average age of 61. All women received a calcium supplement so that their total daily intake including food sources was 800 mg daily. Half of the women received 400 IU of vitamin D and the other half placebo. Over the course of a year the women receiving the additional vitamin D had a significant gain in bone density." Dawson-Hughes B et al. Effect of vitamin D supplementation on wintertime and overall bone loss in healthy postmenopausal women. *Ann Intern Med* October 1, 1991;115(7):505–512.

Page 211 . . . "Studies have shown that low vitamin K is associated with osteoporosis and is important for the healing of fractures. Those with osteoporotic fractures frequently have low blood levels of vitamin K." Bittensky L et al. Circulating vitamin K levels in patients with fractures. *J Bone Joint Surg* 1988; 70-B: 663–664.

Page 212 . . . "Vitamin C deficiency has been shown to cause osteoporosis in animal studies." Hymans et al. Scurvy, megaloblastic anemia and osteoporosis. *Br J Clin Pract* 1963; 117:332–340.

Page 212 . . . "A 1988 inspired great interest when boron supplementation reduced urinary calcium and magnesium excretion, and increased blood levels of estrogen (17-beta estradiol) by 44 percent." Nielsen F. Boron—an overlooked element of potential nutritional importance. *Nutr Today* Jan/Feb 1988; 4–7.

Page 213 . . . "Several double-blind studies have shown that ipriflavone increases bone density when combined with calcium." Agnusedei D, Buffalino L. Efficacy of ipriflavone in established osteoporosis and long term safety. Calcif Tissue Intl, 1977; Suppl 1(61):PS23–27. Gennari C et al. Effect of chronic treatment with ipriflavone in postmenopausal women with low bone mass. *Calcif Tissue Intl* 1992;51 Suppl 1:S30–34. Valente M et al. Effects of 1 year treatment with ipriflavone on bone in postmenopausal women with low bone mass. *Calcif Tissue Intl* 1994;54: 377–380.

Page 213 . . . "One negative study published in the *Journal of the American Medical Association*" reported that ipriflavone combined with calcium was no better than placebo in slowing bone loss." Alexandersen P et al. Ipriflavone in the treatment of postmenopausal osteoporosis. *JAMA* 2001; 285:1482–1488.

Page 213 . . . "Studies have shown that approximately 40 percent of postmenopausal women have low stomach acid." Grossman M et al. Basal and histalog-stimulated gastric secretion in control subjects and in patients with peptic ulcer or gastric cancer. *Gastroenterology* 1963; 45:15–26.

Chapter 12

Page 219 . . . "Since osteoarthritis of the knee is twice as common in women than men, researchers investigated the impact high-heeled shoes have on knee osteoarthritis. They concluded that the altered forces at the knee caused by walking in high heels may in fact predispose to degenerative changes in the joint " Kerrigan DC et al., Knee osteoarthritis and high heeled shoes. *Lancet* May 9, 1998;351(9113):1399–1401.

Page 219 . . . "Canadian researchers found that women who had used synthetic hormones for five years or longer were twice as likely as nonusers to develop osteoarthritis." Wilkins K. Hormone replacement therapy and incident arthritis. *Health Rep* Autumn 1999;11(2):49–57.

Page 219 . . . "An additional study examined the association of synthetic estrogen replacement therapy and the incidence of arthritis." Sahyoun NR, Hochberg MC, Pamuk ER. Estrogen replacement therapy and incidence of self reported physician diagnosed arthritis. *Prev Med* May 1999; 28(5): 458–464.

Page 234 . . . "Propolis is a bee product that proved in one study to be more effective than acyclovir in healing genital herpes lesions." Vynograd N et al. A comparative multi-centre study of the efficacy of propolis, acyclovir and placebo in the treatment of genital herpes. *Phytomedicine* Mar 2000;7(1):1–6.

ABOUT THE AUTHORS

Angela Stengler, N.D., is a popular and respected naturopathic doctor, lecturer, and author. Her expertise in women and children's health makes her a frequent guest of radio and television programs. She is a strong advocate of the role of natural medicine for women's health. She received her Bachelor's Degree from Pitzer College, and her four-year Doctorate of Naturopathic Medicine from the National College of Naturopathic Medicine. Dr. Angela has written several articles and books on women's health and is co-author of *Your Vital Child*. She is the host of a natural health radio show. She enjoys spending time with her two children and being a role model for healthy habits.

Mark Stengler, N.D., is known as The Natural Physician to his patients and audiences. He serves on the subcommittee for the Yale University Complementary Medicine Outcomes Research Project. He is the author of several books including *The Natural Physician's Healing Therapies* and co-author of *Your Vital Child*. He practices at La Jolla Whole Health Medical Clinic.

For more about the authors, see their website at:
www.thenaturalphysician.com

Also by the same author:

The Natural Physician's Healing Therapies

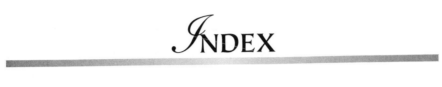

INDEX

N